1994

Beauty is the Beast

Beauty is the Beast

Appearance-Impaired Children in America

Ann Hill Beuf

u/r/r

University of Pennsylvania Press / PHILADELPHIA

Library of Congress Cataloging-in-Publication Data

Beuf, Ann H., 1938–
    Beauty is the beast : appearance-impaired children in America / Ann Hill Beuf.
        p.   cm.
    Includes bibliographical references.
    ISBN 0-8122-8234-5. — ISBN 0-8122-1310-6 (pbk.)
    1. Disfigured children—United States—Sociological aspects. 2. Stigma (Social psychology) I. Title.
HV904.B48 1990
155.9'16—dc20   89-21485
                                                                                          CIP

To my family

HONEY, CARLO, PETER, MAITLAND,

MELINDA, CATHY,

and

MAX

Contents

Acknowledgments

This book is the result of observations made during almost twenty years of sociological research. These observations have been of children with impaired appearance: burns, birth defects, dermatological disorders, weight problems, and eye problems.

The dermatology studies, carried out with my colleague, Professor Judith Porter of Bryn Mawr College, focused specifically on the impact of changed appearance on the social and psychological lives of vitiligo victims. Much of this book is gathered from field notes of research projects which did not have the study of impaired appearance at their core. Nonetheless, during that period a growing amount of my material from studies of hospitalized children, myopic children, and children with eating disorders dealt with the importance of appearance in establishing social relationships and personal self-esteem.

Looking back, I believe that my interest in this matter was first piqued by the late Doctor Kenneth Michaille of Wills Eye Hospital in Philadelphia. While examining my eyes, he asked about my work, and in response to my interest in the social psychology of medicine he described a phenomenon he had observed in children whom he had fitted with soft contact lenses. These elementary- and high-school aged children seemed to experience a "personality change" after getting the lenses, even sitting differently in the office waiting room. While they appeared depressed and shy during their initial visit and sat slumped in their seats, when they returned for the following visit after wearing the lenses for six weeks they sat straight in their chairs and engaged in conversation with other people in the waiting room.

At Dr. Michaille's suggestion, we collaborated on a project that confirmed these impressions. Using interviews, game playing, and the Coopersmith measure of self-esteem, we were able to show the elevation of self-esteem and social interaction that came from discarding "sodapop-bottle-bottom" glasses for invisible contact lenses. We also observed some differences between social groups: girls were more concerned with cosmetic change, boys with the ability to participate in sports; children of different age levels were more or less worried about appearance.

During the early 1970s, I began a study of eating disorders in adolescent and college-age women. During this research, as one pathetic-looking anorexic after another told me of the approval her initial acts of self-starvation had generated, I began to see the importance of cultural beliefs, attitudes, and values in determining how people with "different" appearances are treated.

At this time, I was also studying the ways children are treated in hospitals. The field work for this project brought me into daily touch with children waiting for plastic surgery—children with cleft palates, facial burns, and other deformities.

I served on a United Nations committee for stigmatized children during the United Nations International Year of the Child, 1978. The committee included many respected scholars; hearing their papers and listening to their discourse has enriched the theoretical aspect of this book. The value of working at the intersection of various disciplinary fields had become apparent by this time, too.

I am, therefore, grateful to a large number of people whose friendship and collegiality embarked me on this project. Vitiligo cases in this book are drawn from original research funded by NIH grant #IP50-AM25252-04.

Chapter 1

Introduction

> Would Eleanor Roosevelt have had to struggle to overcome
> this tortuous shyness if she had grown up secure in the
> knowledge that she was a beautiful girl? If she hadn't strug-
> gled so earnestly, would she have been so sensitive to the
> struggles of others? Would a beautiful Eleanor Roosevelt
> have escaped from the confinements of the mid-Victorian
> drawing room society in which she was reared? Would a
> beautiful Eleanor Roosevelt have wanted to escape? Would
> a beautiful Eleanor Roosevelt have had the same need to
> be, to do?
>
> HELEN GAHAGAN DOUGLAS
> *The Eleanor Roosevelt We Remember*

On Monday, March 1, 1988, an American sixth-grade student walked
into his elementary school classroom and shot himself. He did this
because his classmates had teased him about being overweight. When
I read this child's story, I was deeply saddened but not surprised.
Nearly twenty years of working with children who are, in one way or
another, socially stigmatized had convinced me that there is a terrible
psychological price to pay for having an "unacceptable" physical
appearance in our society. Not only do we Americans set narrow
standards of beauty and then insult and hurt those who fall outside
those standards, but our adult society, because of its ambiguous
concept of childhood and children, functions to disempower and
discriminate against children, thus giving them a double stigma to
bear.

Although, as a medical sociologist, I hope that my colleagues will
find some productive thought herein, my major intention is to attract
those who deal with appearance-impaired children. Nurses, child
psychologists, social workers, child life workers and teachers, as well

as parents can find in this material some help in working with children whose appearance is impaired.

There is a need for such an approach, for, while there are some excellent sociological and psychological works on stigma, there is little that deals with *children* and stigma in terms of social, psychological, and medical concepts.

This book is comprised of observations made over nineteen years of working with children with impaired appearance. In some cases these children were not the focus of my research at the time I observed them, but were part of other studies. In some instances, impaired appearance *was* the focus of the research. In all the projects, in-depth interviewing was done with every child. Those children who were hospitalized were observed as well. These methods were not employed with this book in mind, but they serendipitously have presented me with many similar data on children with such diverse appearance-related disorders as burn scars, anorexia nervosa, extreme myopia, facial scars from injuries, cleft palates, and other cranial-facial disorders. Working with Dr. Alan Lerner of Yale Medical School and Dr. Judith Porter of the Sociology Department of Bryn Mawr College on children with skin diseases gave me access to an important patient population. One of these, vitiligo, is a depigmenting disorder in which the death of melanin cells causes the patient to develop patches of snow-white skin which contrast with the color of the normal skin. As far as is known, vitiligo has no other effect on the body; it does not itch or hurt. This gives us a vital opportunity to study a situation in which appearance impairment is the major or only factor and can therefore be studied for its impact in isolation unencumbered by the painful or dysfunctional elements in other populations of disfigurement.

Goals

My goals in writing this book are basically pragmatic. They are:

1. To describe the experiences of children with impaired appearance accurately and vividly enough to raise general consciousness regarding their treatment within our society, and to impress the general public as well as educational and medical professionals with the need for a more sensitive and positive approach to their treatment.
2. To determine systematically the social, psychological, and physiological factors that either alleviate or intensify the impact of impaired appearance on the lives of such children.
3. To develop a means of assessing this impact in individual children.
4. To suggest ways of helping such children and improving their position in our society.
5. To help the parents of appearance-impaired children understand and respond to the special needs of their children and to act as their advocates.
6. To impress on physicians, teachers, and other professionals who work with children of impaired appearance the importance of appearance in the psychological and social lives of children, and thus of the need to take seriously children's concerns about these matters.

In order to portray the experience of appearance-impaired children in America, it is necessary to combine insights from a variety of social, psychological, cultural, and physiological perspectives. This includes a cross-cultural perspective on the manner in which different societies value appearance and where the United States falls in the spectrum of tolerance for stigma, a consideration of the various systems of interaction through which a child moves, and a developmental approach to the function of age as an intervening variable in stigmatization and coping. We must also consider what social and psychological resources children possess and how these help them cope with the experience of stigmatization.

In all these explorations, we must keep in mind two factors:

certain physiological attributes of the stigma itself, especially its severity, visibility, and whether or not it is located on the face; and the general cultural attitude regarding appearance. The United States, as we will see, has a particularly intolerant attitude toward children with impaired appearance because (1) it is basically ambiguous and unfair in its treatment of children in general, and (2) the overall culture is obsessed with narrow standards of beauty that assume tremendous importance in our type of social system.

Chapter Two discusses the research that has been done on the topic of appearance impairment, and reviews the theoretical perspectives that help one understand the impact of appearance-related disorders on children.

Chapter Three examines differences between and within societies concerning appearance, stigmatization, tolerance for difference, and coping tactics. It discusses our own society's attitudes toward the appearance-impaired against the cross-cultural backdrop. In Chapter Four, I note the manner in which strangers, friends, physicians, and family members have reacted to children with impaired appearance. This chapter also considers the extent to which social acceptance and life chances have been limited by social stigmatization. I also note those social and physiological characteristics which are associated with social stigmatization.

Chapter Five takes up the issue of response to social stigmatization, with special attention to the matter of self-stigmatization. I examine the psychological impact of impaired appearance on the children, and discuss the manner in which various coping resources are effective in limiting or preventing the acceptance by the individual of a stigmatized identity.

Chapter Six presents suggestions for subverting the process which creates social discrimination and psychological suffering in people whose only "offense" is their deviation from the American ideal of beauty.

Chapter 2

Perspectives: Stigmatization, Objectification, and Self

> A sociological theory of deviance must focus specifically upon the interactions which not only define behaviors as deviant, but also organize and activate the applications of sanctions by individuals, groups or agencies. For in modern society, the socially significant differentiation of deviants from the nondeviant population is increasingly contingent upon circumstances of situation, place, social and personal biography, and the bureaucratized activities of agencies of control.
>
> John I. Kitsuse,
> "Societal Reaction to Deviant Behavior"

This book is about being an appearance-impaired child in America today. It is the result of almost twenty years of work with children stigmatized in various ways, work done in association with four medical schools and hospitals. The subjects suffer from many disorders such as vitiligo, a depigmentizing disorder which can create a spotted appearance of the skin;[1] psoriasis and acne; cleft palate; obesity; and myopia. They have appearances that are at odds with the American concept of beauty, although the range in the severity of their disfigurement is great.

Since the early part of this century, researchers have been concerned with the difficulties in social interaction encountered by handicapped persons.[2] Studies have examined how "normals" react to the handicapped,[3] including staring at afflicted people on the street,[4] attribution of personality traits to handicapped people based on their condition,[5] distancing of oneself from the handicapped,[6] and hiring discrimination against the handicapped.[7] They have also studied the impact of handicapping on the victims themselves, their changed roles[8] and the effects the handicap has on personality.[9] While such studies are important and have been helpful to me, the fact that many of the subjects of the research have been physically handicapped prevented me from isolating the effects on social interaction and personality of impaired appearance alone. The children I am concerned with are impaired in appearance *only*, with no associated physical or mental handicap.

Nearly twenty years of reading questionnaires, interviewing children and parents, and observing activities in treatment centers both here and abroad have created in me a painful awareness of the social stigmatization of appearance-impaired children in the United States, the burdensome social consequences of this stigmatization for its victims, and the psychological price such stigmatization exacts.

More optimistically, the coping practices employed by these children—their humor, endurance, and resistance to social devaluation—suggested to me the means by which the lives of those who are stigmatized by impaired appearance could be vastly improved in our society.

America worships beauty. The culture stresses highly idealized images of both male and female attractiveness and urges the common citizen to conform to them. The smooth skin, silky hair, straight noses, and dazzling smiles of models in the media set a narrow standard to which all must try to conform. Enormous sums of money are expended in the quest for beauty in the United States. It has been estimated that in 1980 Americans spent $2.6 billion on cosmetics, $1.5 billion on skin preparations, and close to $400 million on diet aids.[10] Money spent at weight loss centers, beauty parlors, and body building clinics and on plastic surgery adds additional millions to the cost of the national quest for an acceptable appearance.

While few can conform to the ultimate definition of beauty as represented by a handful of models and entertainment personalities, it *is* more possible than ever before for most people to present a pleasant or "normal," if not beautiful, appearance. Innovations in pediatric care, dentistry, and plastic surgery can prevent or correct many of the facial disfigurements of bygone times and prevent accidental injuries from leaving permanent scars. Nutritional gains can prevent damage to body form and limbs from malnutrition and vitamin deficiency. Various systems of medical assistance and third-party payment have brought these advances within the grasp of most people in our country.

For this reason the person whose appearance is impaired, who stands out because of obvious flaws or disfigurements, is perceived as a deviant in the United States. In undeveloped or poor countries, where extreme poverty, lack of medical attention, malnutrition and neglect, and the consequences of physical trauma prevail, it is common to see the limp caused by a childhood fall, the bent limbs of malnutrition, the cheek scarred by the untreated injury of several years ago, the face misshapen by improper dental development. But in America such sights are rare. The physically-impaired or disfigured person in America is deviant in two regards: failing to live up to the cultural standard of beauty, and failing to conform to the United States standard of "normal" or unexceptional appearance.

Types of Research

One problem in understanding the situation of children with impaired appearance has been the tendency of the research to fall into different camps, none of which seem to have much communication with the others. Psychologists and psychiatrists have studied the psychological consequences of impaired appearance, but have tended to disregard the social and medical realities with which their subjects live. When I first began this research, I found several studies in which the fears and anxieties odd-looking people experienced when going about their daily activities or meeting new people were believed to be delusions.[11] *Yet, it is a central truth in the matter of impaired appearance that such feelings of the victims are rooted in reality.* Other people *do,* in fact, see them differently and treat them differently.

The psychological school tends to see this stigmatization and the response of the victim in terms of highly individualized characteristics of both parties to the interaction, stressing the psychological state of the labeler (envious, projecting, insecure) and the victim (self-conscious, embarrassed, feeling inferior).[12] The victim who is able to stand up against labeling is also seen by this school through a personality perspective. Resistance to the degradation that objectification can cause is attributed to self-confidence, competence, and strong ego. The role of such *social* factors as the nature of the stigma itself, the social class of the parties involved, and local or national cultural values is ignored.

Another perspective, that of deviance theory, stresses the importance of social values and norms in determining the very nature of deviance itself. According to deviance theorists, no person or condition is inherently deviant, but only those who have been so labeled by their societies.[13] This concept is an important one in understanding both the differential vulnerability to stigma labels and the variety of responses of stigma victims to their conditions. Here, the actual social events, experiences, and social resources emerge as important variables in the study of the disfigured.

Yet, because the nature of the social label "ugly" leads to a definition of the self as categorically deviant or "typed," the responses of the labeled persons to their condition are too often viewed as being exclusively determined by aspects of the label and the labeling process, and not by any characteristics of the appearance impairment itself or by the social and psychological characteristics of the victim. Lofland, for example, sees the outcome of stigmatization as being primarily rooted in the nature and the extent of the specific stigmatizing, while paying only passing lip service to other facts:

> Other things being equal, the greater the *consistency, duration* and *intensity* with which a definition is promoted by others about an Actor, the greater the likelihood that an Actor will enhance that definition as truly applicable to himself.[14]

Yet other things are rarely "equal" in the lives of real people. This is a limitation of deviance theory. Common, everyday observations as well as the biographies of exceptional people alert us to instances in which social reality flies in the face of such reasoning. We all know of persons whose actions testify to the victory of self-esteem and confidence over social stigmatization. Such persons as Frederick Douglass, an escaped slave, and Eleanor Roosevelt, the object of cruel jokes about her appearance, come immediately to mind. On the other hand, medical and sociology journals are filled with examples of people who were unable to stand up to social stigma, even though the stigma was relatively *inconsistent,* of *short duration,* and not very *intense*. Indeed, far more energy has gone into determining the outcome of the stigmatizing experience than has been devoted to the nature of the stigma or label.

I will argue that developmental age, social and psychological resources, visibility of the impairment, general societal attitudes, and circles of social interaction are all important conditions in determining the appearance-impaired child's coping ability. In doing this, it is my intention to bring to the analysis of impaired physical appearance in children the theory and the research findings of both the sociology of deviance and the social psychology of stigma, as well as developmental theory and the notion of coping resources. From deviance theory as it is now understood by sociologists, we can gain an understanding of the stigmatization of the appearance-impaired child by others, and of some aspects of victim response. From the work of those in social psychology and developmental psychology, the effects of stress on the psychological lives of those who experience it can be studied in a more complex fashion. We can achieve greater insight into the labeled person's susceptibility or resistance to the negative consequences of stigmatization.

It is important here to elaborate on my use of the term "deviance." Because of the tendency of former generations of sociologists to apply this term to certain extreme types of persons and behaviors, the public, and indeed some sociologists, tend to associate the term "deviant" with criminals, madmen, and colorful eccentrics. More recent work in the sociology of deviance has shifted attention from specific people or behavioral patterns to the manner in which societies define and treat deviance.[15] This emphasis, combined with general anthropological observations of the varying norms and norm violations in different cultures, has led to the realization that deviance is not inherent in any type of person or any behavior, but is simply "that which society defines as deviant."[16] Thus, even murder, which we might think to be an inherently deviant act, is not always deviant. In times of war, killing is rewarded. It is only "deviant" under conditions that society declares to be deviant. Nor can we say that a person is "deviant" in any absolute sense. The characteristics which distinguish the shaman or healer in many cultures—visionary experience, hallucination—will lead to respect and material success; in the United States a person with these symptoms might well be institutionalized as schizophrenic.

By "deviant," then, we refer to one who has been labeled as such, or "stigmatized." Nor need a person commit any particular deed or manifest any specific behavior to be labeled "deviant." As Schur has noted, occupation of certain statuses or simply *being* a certain way is often sufficient cause for the application of social stigma.[17] Such is the case of those with impaired appearance. These children are viewed as deviants within our society, as has been empirically demonstrated in a number of research investigations. The social process by which a person's appearance is defined as deviant by others can be referred to as "social stigmatization." The manner in which these people are often thought of, discussed, and treated by others is often called "objectification." This term indicates the dehumanizing aspect of stigmatization and is thus a sub-category of stigmatization.[18]

The acceptance of the stigma by the labeled person will be referred to here as "self-stigmatization." By this we mean what Edwin Lemert called the "ultimate acceptance of deviant social status and efforts at adjustment on the basis of associated role" on the part of the victim.[19]

In groundbreaking research,[20] Karen Dion told her subjects (school teachers) a story about a child who goes to school one morning and, seeing a dog on the playground, begins to throw rocks at the animal. She then showed the subjects a picture of the child. Of course, the story was fictional and the children shown in the picture had not really thrown the stones. She showed half the subjects a picture of a handsome child, and the others a picture of a homely, chubby child who looked rather like Pugsly of the Addams Family. Dion then asked the teachers what they thought had happened in the incident. Those who had been shown the handsome child excused his behavior, many of them saying that perhaps something upsetting had occurred in his home prior to his coming to school. Perhaps one of his parents had yelled at him. The rock-throwing was very atypical behavior as he was usually a kind child. On the other hand, those who had been shown the picture of the homely child were quick to state that this was a kind of mean behavior in which he commonly engaged. Negative traits were attributed to the child and much pity expressed for the dog.

Dion and Miller have both found that subjects are more likely to attribute traits of kindness and intelligence to good-looking people than to others. Researchers have also found that better-looking people are thought to have better self-control and competence.[21]

In both physical and social stigma, a set of negative *emotions* is often tied to this set of beliefs. This is true for the physically stigmatized, although we are expected by society to have a sympathetic attitude toward them. The stigmatized person becomes the object of such emotions as anxiety, fear, guilt, hostility, and even hatred on the part of other persons.[22] Erving Goffman pointed out that this phenomenon is at least partly rooted in the violation of interaction norms that occurs when "normals" and the stigmatized confront each other socially. His studies show that most human interaction is based on a set of common assumptions on the part of the interacting parties about what each brings to the interaction and what norms will govern their exchange.[23] For example, in approaching you to begin a conversation, I assume many things. I assume that you can see me coming, that you will hear me speak, and that you will respond. If it becomes apparent to me at some point that you are unable to fulfill any one of these expectations, I find myself in a socially embarrassing situation. It is this embarrassment and the desire to avoid it or be removed from it which Goffman saw as the dynamic behind much of the hostility directed at stigmatized people. As Allport notes, this hostility can run the gamut from antilocution to homicide.[24]

People are more likely to like good-looking people.[25] Good-looking people are also credited with leading better lives by subjects in many studies.[26] Even in situations of psychoanalysis, Barocas and Vance found that counselors judged attractive subjects closer to achieving mental health than their unattractive counterparts.

Grey and Ashmore found that judicial decisions such as length of sentence were influenced by the defendants' degree of attractiveness.[27] Similarly, Schwartz's study of psychotherapists found they were likely to see attractive patients as improving more rapidly than less attractive ones.[28]

A recent study by Sheila Deitz and her colleagues at the University of Virginia Institute of Law, Psychiatry and Public Policy found that men were more likely to attribute blame for a rape to an unattractive woman than to an attractive one.[29]

Studies show that impaired appearance may have a negative impact on interaction with others.[30] The stigmatized are believed to be less talented, less "good," and leading less meritorious lives than the physically attractive.[31]

Nor is it only attitudes which are influenced. Studies also show that teachers, peers, and counselors may actually discriminate against the physically unattractive.[32] One study that attempted to examine the willingness of people to help an ill individual on the subway found that people were less likely to come to the aid of an individual with a facial birthmark than to that of another person of their own age, race, and apparent social class.[33] Kmiecik found that people move on faster when their space (at a city intersection) is violated by an unattractive intruder than by an attractive intruder.[34]

This apparent desire to avoid interaction is typical of another phenomenon, which social scientists have called "social distance."[35] People usually seek to establish some social distance between themselves and the stigmatized. This can take many forms, from the abrupt termination of a conversation to the deliberate crossing of the street to avoid a stigmatized person to the legislated refusal to sit in the same vehicle or restaurant as the stigmatized.[36] Social distancing is usually related to the holding of *beliefs* and stereotypes about the stigmatized group and to the presence of *negative emotions regarding it*.

It is interesting to note that these three components of discrimination against the stigmatized do not invariably go together. For example, a person might feel kindly toward a stigmatized social group and hold no negative stereotypes about its members, but maintain a large social distance because such action is supported or required by the norms of the community. We are familiar with examples of this phenomenon in many areas of the world. Conversely, a person may hold strong negative stereotypes about a group, but find him- or herself in living quarters with a member of the group while in the armed forces or at school or on the job. These observations should be kept in mind later, when we address the ability to bring about change in this area. Nor are the emotions of others unambiguous. Parents of a disfigured child may feel love, guilt, repulsion, and responsibility all at the same time.

Finally, part of the response of the "others" seems to be rooted in psychological as well as social factors. Recent work in race relations and in the sociology of deviance identifies the notion of "categorical perception," the tendency of others to see the stigmatized trait as the stigmatized person's major characteristic and their tendency to respond to that person mainly as a member of the stigmatized category, rather than as an individual.[37] Other aspects of the person are ignored as the stigmatized trait assumes the characteristics of what sociologists refer to as a "master status."[38]

While all people occupy many statuses—daughter, wife, mother, worker, tennis player—some statuses carry more social significance than others. Age, gender, social class, and race are all "master statuses" in American society. A master status is the first thing others "see" in a person; thereafter, they tend to respond to the person solely in terms of this status, rather than in terms of the complex of statuses occupied by the person or the personality traits he or she possesses.[39] Schur states:

> Numerous studies show that when individuals are "seen" in terms of a deviant status and identity (past or present)—be it "criminal," "homosexual," "madman," "prostitute," "drug addict," "cripple," or "retarded," other people's responses to them are heavily influenced by that identification . . . the individual is responded to first and foremost in terms of his or her presumed membership in the devalued category.[40]

This book will demonstrate the means by which impaired appearance constitutes such a master status. We will see that many children with disfiguring conditions experience interactions with others that are stigmatizing in nature.

Objectification

It has been noted by a variety of researchers that a major characteristic of social stigmatization is *objectification*.[41] Schur notes the dehumanizing effects of objectification, which treats people mainly or solely in terms of the "type" or category in which they have been placed by social stigmatization.[42] The concept of objectification originates in the social psychology of race relations, particularly in the work of Gordon Allport, whose definition of prejudice as "antipathy based upon a faulty and inflexible generalization" recognized the placing of people in generalized categories as one of the major difficulties of stigmatization.[43]

Objectification implies more than the application of the label "deviant." It implies the devaluation of its targets to a less-than-human status. In being treated as a member of a category rather than as an individual, those who have been so categorized are deprived of their personhood. When this happens to a person, he or she is responded to by others—especially control agents or those in the "helping" professions[44]—according to some predetermined, routine protocol deemed appropriate for dealing with "cases" in the labeled category. This tendency has been referred to as the "bureaucratization of deviance."[45] Some of the appearance-impaired people in our sample had experienced this phenomenon in their dealings with medical personnel, who related to them as "cases" and "conditions" rather than as persons.

Not all people are equally susceptible to objectification. High social status, political power, age, or charismatic personality traits may protect persons from being labeled, by being themselves "master statuses" that eclipse the importance of the deviant status or threaten the ability of others to apply or to act on that label.[46] In other cases, a more moderate label may be applied by which deviance is not denied but somewhat modified. This concept is illustrated by the saying, "Poor people are crazy, but rich people are eccentric."

Not all the children I observed experienced the same degree of social stigmatization. Quite a few had been subjected only to mild forms of objectification. Much of the time they were treated as "normal people" whose total persona was taken into account by others.

For those with impaired appearance, one contributor to susceptibility to social stigmatization and objectification is visibility. If other people are unaware of the impairment they do not note, label, or interpret the person's appearance as deviant. This suggests that visibility is related to victims' and others' responses mainly through its influence on discrimination.

Severe impairment, especially if it is visible, *is* more likely to be noted and responded to. With respect to discriminatory behavior, as the data in Chapter Three will indicate, the face is of the greatest significance. Even a small disfiguring mark on the face carries with it considerable social significance and may be reacted to by others. Visible impairment of the hands, while not quite so influential, is second only to the face in determining vulnerability to stigmatization.

The ability to hide or disguise impaired appearance is also related to the importance of visibility, as a correlate of discrimination and thus of stigmatization. The effective use of cosmetics, clothing, and accessories (such as hats, dark glasses, and gloves) can prevent stigmatization. (One subject noted, however, that her efforts at disguise became so extreme—long sleeves, gloves, dark glasses, and a hat in the heat of summer—that another label, that of "oddly-dressed person," was applied to her.)

Those who for reason of gender (male), social class (poor), or religion (fundamentalist) are socially denied access to cosmetic use or to certain types of disguising garb are more susceptible to the label of appearance-impaired. Thus, it was not surprising to find that many of the males had suffered as much or more social stigmatization than the females, despite the greater importance attached to female appearance in American society. Because girls are able to cover and disguise disfiguring conditions, they more frequently elude the social definition of deviant appearance.

Some children suffered needless objectification because their parents believed it immoral or inappropriate for a child to wear make-up. The varying degrees of stigmatization and the factors associated with susceptibility and vulnerability to stigma will be discussed in greater depth in a later chapter.

Victims' Responses to Stigma: Self-Stigmatization and Coping

Stigmatization and objectification do not stop outside the victim. People have experienced social and psychological stress as the result of their deviant status. Numerous studies have documented the impact of stigma on the lives of the stigmatized.[47] One woman with a skin disorder wrote to us, "Please let me know what you find about the self confidence of children with this disorder. I know I was left with a damaged sense of my self since adolescence."

How do its victims respond to the situation of stigmatization? In a variety of possible ways. The late Gordon Allport, in discussing "Traits Due to Victimization," wrote:

Ask yourself what would happen to your own personality if you heard it said over and over again that you were lazy, a simple child of nature, expected to steal, and had inferior blood. Suppose this opinion were forced on you by the majority of your fellow citizens. And suppose nothing that you could do would change this opinion because you happen to have black skin. One's reputation, whether false or true, cannot be hammered, hammered, hammered into one's head without doing something to one's personality.

A child who finds himself rejected and attacked on all sides is not likely to develop dignity and poise as his outstanding traits. On the contrary, he develops defenses. Like a dwarf in a world of menacing giants, he cannot fight on equal terms. He is forced to listen to their derision and their laughter and submit to their abuse.

There are a great many things such a dwarf may do, all of them serving his ego defenses. He may withdraw into himself, speaking little to the giants and never honestly. He may band together with other dwarfs, sticking close to them for comfort and for self-respect. He may try to cheat the giants when he can and thus have a taste of sweet revenge. He may occasionally in desperation push some giant off the sidewalk or throw a rock at him when it is safe to do so. Or he may, out of despair, find himself acting the part that the giant expects and gradually come to share his masters' own uncomplimentary view of dwarfs. His natural self-love may under the persistent blows of contempt, turn his spirit to cringing and self hate.[48]

Allport thus suggests that in-group solidarity, withdrawal, militancy, and low self-esteem are all possible responses to the condition of stigmatization. Erving Goffman has set forth similar categories of response in his book, *Stigma*, which deals with adult responses to stigma.

Wright and others have reported reactions which resemble those set forth by Allport:[49] aggression, bravado, overcompensation, acceptance, use of disability for advance, and "succumbing" strategies such as denial, depression, and withdrawal.[50] In particular, work such as that of Pearlin and Schooler on people's ability to cope with stress—of which both impaired appearance itself and the experiences of social stigmatization are prime examples—asserts that certain "coping" resources are of great importance in determining the impact of stigmatization on the lives of people.[51]

To the extent that we gain our self-image from the image that others have of us, the stigmatized child runs the risk of internalizing an image of himself or herself as an inferior human being. Indeed, unattractive persons, particularly women, are expected to develop compensatory traits of "niceness" and to be appreciative of any gesture of kindness shown them by "normals." A study by Ventimiglia shows that the unattractive do, in fact, conform to such expectations. In that experiment, subjects were observed when experimenters performed an altruistic act for them, and their reactions were studied with special attention to expressions of thanks and gratitude. While such variables as gender of the subject alone, gender of the experimenter alone, and setting produced no significant differences in the amount of thanks elicited, an interaction of gender and attractiveness produced significant results. Unattractive females showered their male benefactors with thanks. It would seem that unattractive women, after accumulating some experience with the social world, come to expect very little from it, particularly from men, and are literally "swept off their feet" by the smallest male gesture of courtesy.[52]

In a perplexing study Hobfoll and Penner.m found that graduate students in clinical psychology rated the self concept of attractive persons they saw on a videotape higher than that of unattractive subjects.[53] The study is perplexing because there are two possible interpretations of the data. The first is that clinical psychology graduate students, like everyone else in our society, are more likely to hold a more positive image of and to attribute more positive characteristics to attractive people.

But there is another possible interpretation. That is, that the students were *correct* in their analysis of the interviews and that the attractive "patients" actually do have a better self concept because *society continuously rewards them for their good looks, while meting out the treatment described above to the less beautiful*. Controlled research that holds constant the content of the verbal interview while varying the attractiveness of the patient could shed light on this puzzling phenomenon.

Assorted studies indicate that the impact of stigma on its victims ranges from relatively mild social embarrassment to extreme psychological stress. We might, in fact, say that the ultimate form of objectification occurs when the victims themselves, taking the role of the "others," internalize stigmatized views of themselves. This involves a lowering of the self-image, or what Goffman called "spoiled identity."[54] This is the cruelest price exacted by the process of deviance labeling.

This concept of the devaluation of the victim's self and the attitudes and behavior that arise from the victim's taking a stigmatized view of him- or herself constitute what we shall refer to as *self-stigmatization*. Insofar as the attitudes or actions of the victim can be attributed to realization and acceptance of social stigmatization, we can say that to the corresponding extent their self concept has been altered by stigmatization. Of course, a few exceptional people are able to be aware of social stigmatization and to reject it totally. The different *degrees* of patients' acceptance of stigmatized identities is discussed in Chapter Four. As we shall see, the victim's ability to resist personal devaluation and damaged self concept depends on a variety of factors.

In general, however, social stigmatization has negative consequences for its victims. Schur notes that stigma tends both to punish and to "contain" the stigmatized.[55] It can do this in several ways: by reducing the person's social acceptability, by blocking the person's important social and economic opportunities, and by diminishing the person's overall life chances. As our data indicate, persons with socially stigmatized appearance may experience one, a few, or all of these forms of punishment and containment. Other literature substantiates the reality of the social punishment and control of those with impaired appearance.[56]

Sometimes there are severe psychological consequences to social stigmatization. Some researchers have explored the role of the self-fulfilling prophecy as a response to stigmatization.[57] Attending to others' definition of one's self as deviant, the labeled person internalizes this definition, thus acquiring a deviant self-image. The person then begins to behave in ways that confirm the original definition of deviance. In the case of impaired appearance, a girl might accept society's definition of her as "ugly" or "unattractive" and begin to behave like an "unattractive person." For instance, she might assume a humble, slumping posture, hold her hands in front of her face, and mumble. These behaviors do, in fact, reinforce her "unattractiveness."

Impaired self-esteem has been noted as a result of stigmatization. It is hard to maintain a positive self concept when that self is somehow devalued by others. Because we have all been socialized to value the opinions of others, it is hard for us to deny social definitions even when they are applied to ourselves.[58] Some of the children I have seen have become extremely demoralized by the impairment of appearance. Being viewed as ugly in a society that worships beauty causes people to experience despair, anxiety, and, in some cases, severe depression.

Pearlin and Schooler note three general types of coping strategies:

1. those which change the situation out of which stressful experience arises;
2. those which control the meaning of the stressful experience after it occurs; and
3. those which function for the control of stress after it has occurred.[59]

Applying this set of observations to the situation of impaired appearance, we would recognize the first type of coping strategy in the use of cover-up and disguise material discussed above. That is, the stressful event of social stigmatization can be prevented by hiding impaired appearance from others. This type of coping response can be associated with the prevention or modification of the labeling or social stigmatizing itself.

Once social stigmatization has occurred, the other two types of strategy are called into play. Some disfigured children, as we shall see, employ strategies of the second type. Basically, they attempt to deny or reinterpret social stigmatization after it has taken place, either by denying that it happened in the first place or by attributing its having happened to some deviant characteristic in the stigmatizing agent. Thus, a child might attribute the stares of people on the street to the starers' lack of manners rather than to the child's own appearance.

Most children I observed engaged in a variety of coping behaviors of the third type. That is, after social stigmatization had occurred and they recognized the fact, they attempted to cope with the social conditions and feelings of self-stigmatization that resulted. In this attempt they drew on many sources of support in their social environments and in themselves.

Pearlin and Schooler suggest that these sources of strength can be viewed in terms of two categories of "coping resources": social resources and psychological resources.[60] Distinguishing these coping resources from coping *responses,* Pearlin and Schooler state that while coping response "refers to what people *do* to cope," coping resources are "the resources that are available to them in developing their coping repertoire."[61]

Viewing impaired appearance as a form of stress, we can make productive use of Pearlin's scheme to understand people's responses to stigmatization, because, in addition to observing what people do, we need to comprehend what options and limitations are imposed on individuals and groups of people which set the parameters of the responses actually available to them.

Just as there are varying degrees of susceptibility to social stigmatization (as noted above) that are dependent on such factors as race, social class, or visibility, so is there a range of vulnerability and resistance to self-stigmatization. The ability of the stigmatized person to prevent the negative social and psychological consequences of stigmatization and objectification lies in the nature and extent of the coping resources at his or her disposal.

Social resources are located in a person's social network. They represent potential sources of support. A strong family, compatible fellow workers, or members of one's religious congregation can all help a person cope with stigmatization.[62] *Psychological* resources can be viewed as "the personality characteristics that people draw upon to help them withstand threats posed by events and objects in their environment."[63] Such strengths as high self-esteem, feelings of competency, and the ability to maintain a sense of humor can be effective tools in coping. *Personality traits* such as high self-esteem, humor, and intelligence are also coping resources.[64]

One would predict that those with such coping resources would be less vulnerable to self-stigmatization than those with fewer, weaker resources.

High socio-economic status is a coping resource. The stigmatized person of means will be afforded more protection than the poorer one. If physical stigma is the problem, wealthy families can afford the finest in medical technology to improve the person's appearance or provide training in compensatory skills. Such a family will be less subject to teasing and discrimination, and thus to feelings of incompetence. No matter what the physical appearance, the child of a noble, religious leader, or wealthy businessperson has "borrowed prestige" derived from the parent's position in society and will be treated with the same respect. Poor people, on the other hand, will suffer doubly, as stigmatized people and as poor people. The disrespect and contempt so often demonstrated toward the poor is magnified by the presence of stigma.

A Model for Understanding Children and Stigma

This review of the literature, as well as my observations of and talks with appearance-impaired children, has suggested that a very complex approach is required in order to assess the social and psychological condition of each impaired child.

SOCIO-CULTURAL SYSTEM

First, we must consider the general socio-cultural system, the macro-system in which the child lives. How concerned with appearance are its people? What are the standards of beauty and deviance? How are the unbeautiful treated? We might think of this as the "social backdrop" to all the other factors we must consider. A child with facial deformity in a society which pays much attention to spiritual matters will have an advantage over one with the same disorder in a society preoccupied with beauty. Similarly, children who live in a society with ample and free medical technology to correct their impaired appearance surgically may fare better than in a less advantaged system or one in which access to medical care is determined by material wealth.

Once the overall socio-cultural backdrop has been established and described, we must consider several other factors in assessing the child's condition.

DEVELOPMENTAL AGE

Ironically, given the popularity of developmentalism in western psychology, little has been written about developmental stages as factors in children's response to stigma. Yet, common sense alone would suggest the importance. Surely the adolescent will take disfigurement harder than a five-year-old!

PHYSIOLOGICAL FACTORS

Of primary importance are the realistic parameters of appearance established by the nature of the impairment itself.

1. *Visibility.* How obvious is the impairment to others? Children with visible impairment will experience more stigmatizing events, as other people notice them more than they do children with less visible conditions. Yet *fear of exposure* is a problem for children with hidden stigma.
2. *Severity.* How widespread is the impairment? An impairment can be visible but minor. One facial blemish or scar is visible, but the visible flaw is not always widespread (as in acne on the entire face). The more severe the problem, the more stigmatiz-

ing experiences, and thus stress, are experienced by the child. Intervening variables can modify responses, however.

3. *Repairability*. Does the condition have a bio-medical or surgical resolution? The child whose appearance can in fact be improved is likely to fare better than one for whom such forms of intervention are as yet unknown, or for whom they are too dangerous. While many surgical techniques now in existence can vastly improve the appearance of some forms of cleft lip and palate, neurofibromatosis, the disorder which plagued John Merrick, "The Elephant Man," is in many cases untreatable, because the tumors involve and become entangled with vital parts of the neurological system, which might themselves be damaged in a surgical effort.

Pain. While I attempt in this book to isolate the effects of impaired appearance alone, we must not forget that, in many instances, appearance impairment is associated with pain and dysfunction. These are certainly deficits when it comes to coping, as they may interfere with the child's ability to develop a sense of personal competency and effectiveness, and in general may drain the child's stamina and energy and contribute to feelings of depression or withdrawal.

PSYCHOLOGICAL RESOURCES

Children's humor, self-esteem, intelligence, creativity, and enthusiasm are all important weapons in the arsenal against despair. Such traits permit the child to place other concerns and interests above concern with the impairment, to concentrate on achievement, and to cope with stigmatizing incidents when they occur. Those lacking such resources are the most likely victims of self-stigmatization.

SOCIAL RESOURCES

Such factors as high economic status, high parental status in the community, ethnic group support, parental education, and political power are assets. Ignorance, poverty, low status, lack of education, and social isolation are detrimental. Family support and solidarity are pulses. Psychological, mental, and physical impairment of a parent are minuses. Transitions intensify the reaction to stigmatization.

LEVELS OF INTERACTION WITH THE SOCIAL SYSTEM

One reason it has been difficult to assess the impact of stigma on children is that they move constantly through different levels of the same system—from the privacy of their own room and thoughts to the family circle to the neighborhood and the community. A child may do well at one of these levels but not at others.*

Figure 1 is a visual representation of this model. I shall follow the model in my analysis of appearance impairment, throughout this book, beginning in Chapter Three with a discussion of the cultural backdrop.

*This fact may also help explain some of the differing conclusions of research on this topic. A child interviewed alone, at home, may present a well-adjusted picture; but the same child, questioned at school in the company of peers, might present an entirely different one.

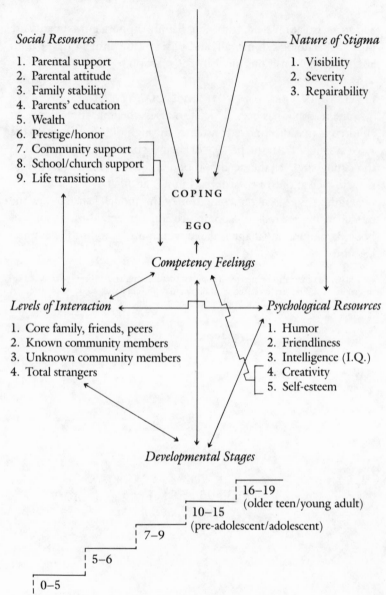

Overall Cultural Attitudes

Social Resources

1. Parental support
2. Parental attitude
3. Family stability
4. Parents' education
5. Wealth
6. Prestige/honor
7. Community support
8. School/church support
9. Life transitions

Nature of Stigma

1. Visibility
2. Severity
3. Repairability

COPING

EGO

Competency Feelings

Levels of Interaction

1. Core family, friends, peers
2. Known community members
3. Unknown community members
4. Total strangers

Psychological Resources

1. Humor
2. Friendliness
3. Intelligence (I.Q.)
4. Creativity
5. Self-esteem

Developmental Stages

16–19
(older teen/young adult)

10–15
(pre-adolescent/adolescent)

7–9

5–6

0–5

FIGURE 1. Factors in Coping Ability

Chapter 3

The Cultural Backdrop

> Down through the ages the experiences of childhood have
> been as varied as its duration. Actions that would have pro-
> voked a beating in one era elicit extra loving care in an-
> other. Babies who would have been nurtured exclusively by
> their mothers in one epoch are left with day-care workers
> in another. In some places children have been taught to
> straddle unsteady canoes, negotiate treacherous mountain
> passes, and carry heavy bundles on their heads. In other
> places they have been taught complicated concerti and long
> multiplication tables.
>
> Barbara Kaye Greenleaf,
> *Children Through the Ages,* p. iv

The previous chapter presented a model that allows us to assess the
child's ability to respond to impaired appearance (Figure 1). We saw
that social and psychological resources, level of social interaction, and
the physiological aspects of the impairment all play roles in determining the child's ability to cope. At the top of the diagram, over-arching
all these factors, is the general nature of the cultural system within
which the child must live. A powerful system of beliefs, attitudes, and
values, the culture of each human society provides a world-view for its
inhabitants that ensures the development of a sense of right and
wrong, good and bad, and instills these in its citizens. It usually affects
and is affected by other parts of the social system. The cultural
attitudes and beliefs about impaired appearance will partly determine
how children with impaired appearance are treated by providing the
general backdrop before which the human drama of stigmatization is
played out.

Thus, regardless of the other variables with which we will work, and which set one child's response off from those of others, American twentieth-century culture is one factor that all the children share. It is what distinguishes American children's experience from that of children in other societies and even from that of American children of the eighteenth or nineteenth century.

This culture contains many elements that can make life hard for appearance-impaired children: a narrow standard of beauty, a mate selection process that stresses physical attractiveness, an ambivalent attitude toward children in general. Fortunately, it also contains factors of a more positive nature: the Judeo-Christian ethic of tolerance, and the heterogeneity of the population, which makes it possible to appreciate more than one type of beauty.

In this chapter, we shall examine the cultural backdrop of American society and some of its impacts on the lives of children with impaired appearance. Information about cultures other than our own will be noted from time to time to set the characteristics of American culture in bold relief, but this is not a cross-cultural analysis in the usual sense of the word. Rather it is an attempt to view American treatment of the appearance-impaired from a global, non-ethnocentric perspective.

Although it seems that every human society places *some* value on what it regards as "normal" or "beautiful" appearance and stigmatizes other appearances, human cultural groups show considerable variation in how important they think appearance is, in what comprises a "normal" or "abnormal" appearance, in how universal its appearance standards are, and in its responses to impaired appearance.

Some societies are relatively unconcerned about what people look like. The !Kung bushmen of the Kalahari Desert, who work cooperatively to hunt animals and gather roots, are reported to value character traits over physical appearance. Women look for a skilled hunter with a good sense of humor; men value a good disposition in women.[1]

The present regime in China alleges that the problem of stigma is a social construct brought about by the "decadent" Western capitalist emphasis on things superficial. To the Western visitor they quote ancient fables, the gist of which is, "You can't judge a book by its cover."

A few years ago, passing through a burn unit in Beijing with my doctor-hosts, I saw a man whose entire face had been blown off in an industrial explosion, I expressed concern about his psychological state, after being told that he was recovering well physically. My hosts told me that such problems do not exist in China because people are judged not by their looks but by their character. It is the Western obsession with appearance, he told me, that creates despair in *our* disfigured people. People in China do not place beauty above all else.

However, things are not always so simple as they seem. Consider my field notes on that encounter in October 1983:

I asked a doctor in the burn unit about the psychological aspects of the severely-burned man who has no facial features left. He said there is no need to make a "formal" psychological effort in this case. He said that the reason for distress in an American patient in such a situation is that our society would be too concerned with superficial appearance, while their society values deeper things, such as character. Chinese people are not stigmatized on the basis of appearance. Therefore, this burn victim will be accepted by others and not experience psychological stress. In fact, he will be happy. His work unit had selected a bride for him and they were married in the ward last week. The work unit has also found him an appropriate new job and an apartment equipped with many aids for his handicaps. The doctor made no mention of the new wife's feelings in this matter. I asked if it was his belief that all psychological problems come from such external factors. Couldn't the victim's own thoughts and fears about his appearance cause psychological distress? The doctor acknowledged that this might be possible but added that if it *did* happen there was no need to summon psychiatric help as "all doctors learn how to deal with such things in a medical school course called 'Medical Virtue.'"

One of my colleagues asked another doctor if all these theories also applied to female burn patients and was told that females with burns of the face *often attempt suicide,* as they are not considered marriageable. (I guess *their* work units aren't so lucky in arranging marriage!)

Observation: The doctor with whom I had this discussion had a very bad case of the depigmenting disease vitiligo on his face and I noticed that, while he was speaking to me on the lack of "superficial concern with appearance in China," he attempted to keep the affected area of his face entirely covered with his hand.

All human societies care about looks. However, there are a virtually endless variety of concepts of beauty and ugliness on the planet. While Americans are face and figure oriented, Japanese suitors focus on the nape of the neck of the beloved. Other societies emphasize the shape of the feet. Thus, we can see that even *which body parts* are taken into consideration in evaluating appearance is culturally determined.

Even when focusing on the same body features, two societies may hold opposite ideas of beauty. Both Americans and many African cultures think that a woman's waistline is very important. But while Americans think it should be small, not so the members of some of these African groups. Hilde Bruch cites Cloete's "I Speak for the African" with regard to the desirability of fatness in some African countries: "What is his heart's desire? Fat above all things. To be fat himself, to have a fat wife and children and fat cattle." Bruch tells us that "Even before anthropologists made their detailed studies, ancient travellers had reported the curious customs of primitive cultures. In many parts of the African continent young girls at puberty were sent to fattening houses to make them ready for marriage."[2]

Some East African women stretch their lips; Maoris tattooed their faces. For centuries, the young girls of China's upper classes endured the cruel practice of foot-binding, which kept their feet only a few inches long and rendered them so helpless that they had to be carried from room to room by servants.

Even within the same society, concepts of beauty may change with time as fads come and go. In the 1890s, Americans appreciated the full-figured "hour-glass look," while in the 1970s, the anorexic or "Twiggy" look found favor. Long straight hair is "in" one year, curly hair the next. But this is usually a minor variation on some fairly inflexible underpinning. Straight noses and good teeth are *always* "in" in the United States, though the color and style of hair or the shade of lipstick may vary.

Homogeneity versus heterogeneity of standards of appearance within the same society must also be examined. A society comprised of people all of the same ethnic and cultural background usually has a single standard of beauty, as in Japan, or in eighteenth-century England. However, in societies comprised of a variety of peoples, different cultural groups may have standards of appearance which differ from one another.

One unfortunate aspect of human conflict and the oppression and exploitation of some groups by others has been what we might call the "colonialization of beauty," that is, the establishment of one group's standard of beauty as a *universal* standard by which *all* are judged.

Although today we see proud Black children who say "I'm black and I'm beautiful," we must remember that this is a new phenomenon. As recently as the 1950s, a universal concept of American beauty prevailed based exclusively on such Anglo-Saxon traits as fair skin, blue eyes, thin lips, and narrow noses. Members of minority groups were urged to strive for this look through the purchase and application of such products as skin bleaches and hair straightener. Advertisements for these products still appear in publications aimed at third world populations. In the 1960s, women from Korea, Viet Nam, and the Philippines were so influenced by the Western concept of beauty that they subjected themselves to surgery to "round" their eyes.

Within a highly heterogeneous society, one is likely to find several competing concepts of appearance. In Australia, the full-figured, Sophia Loren image prevails in the Italian communities, the fair-haired, thin Anglo in the British groups, and, for both of these, there is also the Aboriginal notion of correct appearance. However, this diversity need not necessarily imply a greater tolerance for *impaired* appearance.

Universality of Definitions

In addition we must consider how well-published and accepted the definitions of "normal" and "beautiful" are in the society. The development of mass media, particularly the visual ones—movies and television—permits the rapid and nearly-total dissemination of a very specific concept of "good appearance" and its violation. Therefore, impaired appearance is more obvious, more categorized, and more agreed upon by more people in such societies.

A "bottom line" of normality seems to exist, regardless of variety. A society may tolerate differing notions of "lovely," but the norms of groups are not stretched to include such anomalies as cleft palate, mottled skin, or missing limbs.

This leads us to a consideration of two of the factors that give a society a high or low level of tolerance for impaired appearance: the degree of medical technology available to correct or prevent impaired appearance and the religious or secular value system of the culture.

Values have been called our "blueprints for behavior."[3] Values keep us on track. Internalized by the vast majority of a population, they motivate us to behave in a predictable and approved way. They bind us to one another and to our social groups.

Groups differ in values they hold about appearance, but they are usually related to beliefs held about appearance. For instance, if a group believes, as did people in nineteenth-century England, that odd appearance is a sign of mental illness, then people who are at odds with appearance norms may be shunned, ridiculed, even put away. Elaine Showalter writes: "In England, Maudsly urged prospective husbands to scrutinize their future wives for "physical signs . . . which betray degeneration of stock . . . any malformation of the head, face, mouth, teeth or ears. Outward defects and deformities are the visible signs of inward and invisible faults which will have their influence in breeding." These deadly females, however, could be readily detected by their large jaws, short arms, "badly shaped heads," large, projecting ears, and flat foreheads.[4]

If no particular meaning is attributed to impaired appearance, greater tolerance toward the odd-looking is found. For example, many cultures revere the aged. Gray hair and a wrinkled face denote the wisdom acquired over a lifetime. However, in our own society, these characteristics are devalued, and associated by many with "witches." Children often believe that an older woman is a witch because of her appearance.

Generalized values are also important in determining people's treatment of the stigmatized. For example, the general Judeo-Christian ethic of "do unto others as you would have them do unto you" has been vital in campaigns to win better treatment for people of unusual appearance in the Western world. Yet, at the same time, the Western European values of scientific curiosity and progress have legitimized the exploitation of such people. The "Elephant Man," John Merrick, was exhibited by his physician, who had condemned the "freak shows" for exploiting Merrick. Of course, he himself exploited Merrick by displaying him in the halls of medicine.

In highly sophisticated Western societies, plastic and orthopedic surgery, dental surgery, orthodontics, and a host of medical and therapeutic advances have created a situation in which disfigurement is rare. Quick responses to burns and lacerations, nutritional gains over diseases that twist the body, the use of orthodontics to rectify facial irregularities—all these make it possible for *most* people in a society to look fairly normal. On the other hand, in primitive societies, unattended disfigurement is quite common. Toothlessness is surely not a rare sight in many parts of Africa; nor is hump back, or deformation from accidents and burns, warfare, or injury inflicted by animals. Being so common, it draws less attention than in societies where such sights are rare.

Another social factor influencing the impact of impaired appearance (usually on girls) is the society's method of mate selection or courtship. If marriages are arranged by the parents for such practical reasons as the acquisition of land or power, the bride's appearance may count very little in the evaluation of her assets. Or, in many agrarian societies, the girl's strength, health, and cooking skills may far outweigh beauty. However, in a society such as that of the high-ranking castes of nineteenth-century India, the bride's unblemished beauty was very important, and a scar or skin lesion was enough for the groom's family to call off the betrothal. In Western culture, most marriages are based on romantic choice and appearance is of great importance.

There are also within-society differences that tend to magnify or diminish the attention given impaired appearance. Ugliness is rarer in the upper classes that can usually afford to repair it—or may even possess sufficient power to redefine "beauty" in a way more favorable to its own members. For example, in the United States, upper class, thin women are called "svelte" rather than "scrawny" and others are urged to emulate them.

An example of this is the high prestige accorded girls with braces in posh schools along Philadelphia's prestigious Main Line. Several years ago, the "social pacesetters" in the fifth grade in one school all found themselves weighted down with orthodontic metal. In the past, this had been considered "ugly" or embarrassing. However, once the balance tipped and the majority had braces, *and* once it was learned that the cost of this ordeal was right up there with that of a BMW, wearing braces became a status symbol. Those who did *not* get braces were looked down upon. Several girls asked their parents to "get them braces," out of fear of being ostracized.

Cultural Consistency

One important factor in determining the persuasiveness of a cultural theme or ideology is the degree to which *all* aspects of the culture are consistent in the message they convey concerning this theme or ideology. The fewer contradictions there are in society regarding a cultural theme, the more power it gains. For example, an idea which is agreed upon by theologians, doctors, lawyers, the media, and important political figures has more power than an idea over which these parties disagree. When there is total unanimity among culture purveyors concerning an idea or theme, psychologist Daryl Bem contends that a "non-conscious ideology" exists.[5]

In American society in the late twentieth century, a non-conscious ideology exists regarding thinness. Thinness is seen as beautiful, moral, normal, mature, and healthy. Thinness is supported by aesthetics, psychology, medicine, theology, and the mass media. Both the cultural approval given for weight loss and the social rewards for starving behavior function to (1) increase the number of emotionally disturbed people who employ undereating behavior as a vehicle for the expression of their pathology; and (2) increase the number of otherwise undisturbed people who, in an effort to conform to cultural norms of beauty, engage in undereating behavior. Until recently no countervailing body of theory or information has existed that negates the value or healthiness of thinness. Since the ideology of thinness is so pervasive in our culture, it will be useful for us to take a closer look at the elements that comprise it.

THINNESS IS BEAUTIFUL

Despite a long Western tradition of heavy, beautiful women (from Michelangelo's models to Sophia Loren), emphasis on slimness as an essential ingredient of female attractiveness has characterized American concepts of beauty for most of this century. This emphasis is readily discernible in a consideration of women's magazines, advice columns and advertisements. It is tied to social class as well, with the rich tending to be more slender than the poor. Thus, the young woman believes she can attain a measure of status as well as attractiveness by becoming and remaining slim. It has been said that "You can't be too rich or too thin."

Because 90 percent of anorexics are female, perhaps a note on sex-role differences in this context is in order. Women more than men tend to be evaluated for their beauty and sex appeal. They have always been subjected to ridiculous extremes in the name of fashion, from Scarlett O'Hara corsets to the Twiggy look to the lethal platform shoes of the 1970s. Further, women are expected to subject themselves to a variety of painful experiences—from foot binding to plastic surgery—in order to achieve beauty.

We can document changes in anorexia nervosa following changes in the ideals promoted. A student, Rysella Dgulash, and I tracked the shapes of the "ideal woman" in magazines in the United States from the 1890s to the 1980s. Until the mid-1920s, full-figured womanhood was glorified. Models in clothing advertisements are "matronly"; they appear to be in their late twenties and their thirties and of a moderate weight. (Some even appeared quite fat to 1980s researchers.) In the late 1920s, flappers' clothing became more revealing (skirts were above the knee) and the emphasis shifted to flat-chested youthfulness. The models appear to be in their early twenties and are much more slender than the earlier models. From the mid-1930s to the 1950s, fashion played up the "sexiness" of the woman. Models from this period were in their twenties and thirties, of moderate weight, slim-waisted but quite full-bosomed. Betty Grable and Jane Russell were the "pin-up" girls of World War II. The 1960s and early 1970s gave rise to the skinny, long-legged teen-aged model with little or no bust. The "Twiggy" look was in.

The times when anorexia has proliferated have followed a cultural emphasis on slimness. In the late 1920s, on the heels of the "flapper era," when slenderness was stylish, came a major "outbreak" of the disorder. In the 1970s and 1980s the incidence increased dramatically following the introduction of extremely thin models.

THINNESS IS MORAL—PROTESTANT/FREUDIAN ABSTENTIONISTS

It is certainly no novel observation that our culture has been substantially influenced by the Protestant ethic. The heavy emphasis on self-denial and asceticism that characterized the Puritans has filtered into the mainstream of twentieth-century American culture. Such traits have become synonymous with "goodness" and "morality." The thin person, by his or her very appearance, seems a walking testimony to a life lived in moderation, void of self-indulgence. By comparison, the heavier person is viewed as self-indulgent and lacking in will power.

Even the recent secularization of our society has done little to disabuse people of these beliefs, because modern psychiatry, the "scientific religion" of our times, maintains them. Instead of being viewed as righteous, the thin person is now seen by the psychologically-oriented as "mature" and free of "oral hang-ups," while the heavy person is diagnosed as poorly adjusted or mentally disturbed.

There are, assuredly, important theoretical differences between Protestantism and psychology, but in experiential terms, concerning eating behavior, these may not make too much difference. Whether seen by Puritans as morally upright or by Freudians as "mature egos," thin persons are regarded favorably. Whether seen by Puritans as "immoderate sinners" or by Freudians as beset by oral hang-ups, heavier persons are suspect.

THINNESS IS HEALTHY—NUTRITIONAL FADS

The period since the 1960s has been characterized by an emphasis on weight loss as a preventive measure in the control of such diseases as heart conditions, diabetes, and hypertension. Thus, in the interest of good health, Americans have been urged to abstain from sugar, to use cholesterol-containing food with extreme moderation, and, above all, to reduce their caloric intake.

In addition, the youth culture has been much taken with the health food movement, which stresses the use of all natural ingredients, implying that the preservatives used by the large manufacturers are literally poison to the human system. Vegetarianism also has had an impact on the young.

Many of the precautions of diet and exercise that doctors have urged us to observe are undoubtedly wise; however, there is reason to believe that they have been taken to extremes in our society. Anorexia is not the only alternative to obesity. There is also *normal weight* as a third and highly desirable option. Yet this third alternative is virtually ignored in the cultural emphasis on thinness. Nutrition and a balanced diet are rarely stressed in either medical or popular media. This emphasis manifests itself in the popular culture as well, in the fad diets and starvation techniques suggested by magazines and newspapers.

One of the anorexic girls I interviewed went from 140 to 70 pounds, while working in her doctor-father's office. This man casually looked on as his child lost one half of her total body weight in three months, stating that it was a "good example" for his patients!

Thus, to well-established *evaluative* images of the thin woman as desirable and moderate, we have, in this century, seen the emergence of the *cognitive* belief in the thin person as healthy in mind and body. A non-conscious ideology of thinness as beautiful, moral, and healthy prevails. Yet objectively, extreme thinness, like obesity, is rife with the potential for damage to health, psyche, and the quality of life. Anorexia has one of the highest mortality rates of any behavioral/psychological disorder.

SOCIAL REWARDS

As a result of the unmitigated positive value placed on thinness and weight loss, advertisements for weight loss pills, devices, and programs do not promise only weight loss but a "new life"—friends, romance, affection. In *Such a Pretty Face,* Millman reports that in the Weight Watchers program losers are rewarded with effusive praise while non-losers are ridiculed.[6] This pattern demonstrates the force of a non-conscious ideology in society.

Lack of Support in Social Institutions

Coincident with cultural emphasis on beauty, we often find that the state, the schools, and the medical establishment operate against the needs of the stigmatized. Even family can be rejecting. This lack of support can manifest itself in both direct and implicit ways.

1. The state may have policies which operate against the stigmatized. Health insurance policies that perpetuate stigma when the potential exists to correct it may compound the problem unnecessarily. For example, many U.S. insurance companies refuse to cover plastic surgery—maintaining that it is "merely a luxury." At the time, I was studying severely myopic children, the Commonwealth of Pennsylvania Department of Welfare would purchase ugly, thick, breakable spectacles for the children, but would not pay for soft contact lenses that improved their appearance and granted them greater freedom of movement.

2. The medical profession has been slow to acknowledge the great importance of appearance in the evaluation of the self (see Chapter Four). In our study of patients with vitiligo skin disease, Dr. Porter and I found that there is a tendency for doctors to trivialize such conditions, reminding the patients that worse luck could have befallen them.

Unexpected psychological results of medical therapeutic measures seem to surprise physicians. For example, in reviewing the results of earlier facial surgery on child-patients, Murray, Mulliken, Kapan, and Belfer observe that an improvement of body-image as measured by the Draw-a-Man test occurred in at least one patient.[7] Salyer *et al.* report:

> As satisfaction has been high as judged by the patients, surgeons and psychiatrists. . . . The benefits of early operation on growth and function are not surprising: however, *the favorable improvement in body image has been unanticipated and gratifying.*[8] (Emphasis mine.)

3. Families differ in the amount of support they give their members. Some reject the stigma and may fail to provide the child with a sense of pride. Others take a positive role, providing support with positive attitudes. In the case of the handicapped or disfigured child, parental guilt and shame may cause rejection of the child, who then feels abandoned in an unfriendly world.[9]

4. Even the churches transmit double messages about appearance. Stressing attention to what lies beneath the surface and preaching kindness to the unfortunate transmit one message. Yet all too often, in its Western ethnocentrism and inflexibility, the church has associated a certain kind of appearance with righteousness. Sunday school lessons, for instance, depict "good" women like Ruth and Esther as pretty, and "bad" women, like Lot's wife, as ugly. Of course it is assumed that the Almighty is beautiful. In the 1960s, many white people were shocked when the possibility was raised of Christ having been black. Feminists have suggested that the Deity may be female. Contemplate, if you will, how the suggestion might be received that Jesus was "funny-looking." That contemplation should serve to remind us of the strength of traditional cultural images.

The Status of Children in Society

To understand more fully the situation of the child with impaired appearance, we must understand not only how the society feels about appearance, but also how it feels about children in general.

In pre-industrial societies, children are highly valued, primarily because they play productive economic roles. In hunting, fishing, and farming cultures, children are a vital resource. However, with industrialization, the child becomes an expenditure—an economic consumer who does not produce.[10] The birth rate drops, and the view of the child shifts. Children are seen as more incomplete and less competent in these societies than in pre-industrial groups.

Furthermore, childhood is extended with industrialization. In sixteenth-century France, childhood virtually ended at six years of age. At six, the church confirmed, betrothal took place, and one's economic role began. There were eight-year-old bishops, kings, musicians, and crusaders. The seven-year-old and the seventy-year-old alike had very few rights in feudal Europe, but they had a fairly equal status.[11] In industrial societies, on the other hand, sharp distinctions are made between adults and "children." "Childhood" now lasts into the twenties. Furthermore, in most industrialized democracies, the rights automatically extended to adults are denied to children. Not considered a "person" under the law, the child is relegated to the status of a thing possessed by others.[12] Just who is believed to own the child may vary—in Russia it is the state, in Germany the parents—but the child is the property of *others* and the legal systems of Western industrial societies treat the child accordingly. The 1987–88 case of "Baby M" illustrates this point. Because of his wife's fear that a pregnancy would injure her health, a man arranged for his sperm to fertilize the egg of another woman who carried the fetus throughout pregnancy and delivered the infant. After the birth, this woman decided that she wanted to keep the infant, although she had signed a contract in which she agreed to relinquish the child to the couple in exchange for a monetary fee. The couple alleged that they were the true parents and counter-sued for custody. This entire affair illustrates the objectified status of the child as a piece of property: the original "purchase" of the child from the surrogate mother, the failure of the first court to give much weight to the baby's needs over those of the adults, and the eventual decision, which rested not so much on what the best interest of the baby might be, as on the precedents of *contract law*. That is, the possession of the infant is determined by the nature of the original contract; having promised delivery and taken the money, the surrogate mother is obligated to relinquish the infant just as she would be obligated to relinquish an antique table or ten acres of Wyoming farmland.

Another aspect of the status of children in industrial societies is that, no longer workers or producers but expensive luxuries, they are expected to perform another, subtle role. They are used as display cases for the goodness or success of their families. A well-dressed child testifies to the financial accomplishments of his or her parents, an intelligent child to their brains, a happy child to their kindness. Should the child fail in any of these areas, it is a disgrace to the parents.

When we apply these observations to the situation of appearance-impaired children in contemporary America, we can suggest some hypotheses regarding their treatment by others.

While paying lip service to an appreciation of deeper concerns, we are extremely biased toward beauty, as the literature discussed in Chapter Two indicates. More important, the literature shows us the unfortunate tendency in American society to make associations between appearance and other completely unrelated characteristics. Beautiful people are believed to be *better people*—kinder, more generous, brighter—than others. Homely people have traits such as cruelty, miserliness, bullying attributed to them by people who have never met them.

Our folklore reflects the basic contradiction between a *caveat* to be kind to the stigmatized and our dread and loathing of ugliness. Fairy tales such as the tale of the frog prince (who can only be liberated by the princess's kiss) or "Beauty and the Beast" contain both themes. A nationally televised version of the latter shows the Beast as a deformed man who lives under the city of New York, helping crime victims. Beauty, a "beautiful" yuppie female, loves him, but he must remain where all such ugly creatures, past and present, have lived—in the nether world of darkness—an underworld exile. Movies and novels also reflect this duality. The instant success of the Broadway musical "The Phantom of the Opera" testifies to it.

For the child who "looks different" in our society, this duality is a vise in which he or she is trapped.

American institutions, as noted above, are also less than 100 percent supportive. Insurance policies and health programs that will fund purely "medical" problems may refuse payment for "cosmetic" difficulties, such as plastic surgery to alter disfigurement. I have seen many children whose desire to hide a disfigurement with clothing or make-up has been thwarted by a needless school policy. For example, one child hid a patch of white hair with a hat. A teacher refused to help him and insisted that he remove the hat. Of course, he was ridiculed by classmates. Nor has the educational institution done much within its own classrooms to better the attitudes of "normals" toward the appearance-impaired, or to make the affected child more comfortable with his or her condition.

American culture loves and hates its children. We talk about how much we love them; we spend incredible sums of money on them, and, at least in the white upper and middle classes, we agonize over their psyches. Yet we abuse them—and at an ever-increasing rate.[13] We give them many years of schooling, but we are not sure about how good this education really is. We hire interior decorators to "do" their rooms, but have an infant mortality rate far above that of most other industrial countries.

At the macro level of structural analysis, we also see contradictions. Again there is verbal expression of the importance of children from Capitol Hill and the Oval Office, but budget allocations to education and health and welfare are dwarfed by those to defense and other areas; there is also continued disenfranchisement of children through a double standard of justice that fails to grant them full constitutional rights and treats them as property in judicial matters of adoption and other custody decisions.

I have written extensively on this topic elsewhere and do not wish here to belabor the point of children's helplessness in our society.[14] What I do want to make clear is that being a child in our society means that one's options are limited and, therefore, being an appearance-impaired child in America means something different from being an appearance-impaired adult. One's behavior is limited by the many rules and regulations imposed by an adult world, from the written law to school regulations to family custom. For instance, the physically stigmatized adult has the option to hide away like the "Phantom." Researchers working with disfigured adults find that this is not an uncommon form of adaptation. By taking such at-home jobs as telephone solicitor the person can support him- or herself, call in a grocery order to the local store, and pay someone in the neighborhood to pick up and deliver it, and, quite simply, become a recluse. This option is not open to a child with the same disfigurement, because our laws dictate that, if intellectually able, he or she must spend a certain number of years in the school system.

It is interesting to note that *parents* may choose the seclusion tactic for the child. This strategy is seen frequently in Latin cultures where the child's disfigurement is a cause of shame for the *father*. MacGregor cites a case where the child was secluded and hidden until well into his teens.[15]

Another way in which the adult may respond to stigmatic conditions is through the use of dress and cosmetics to hide or disguise the condition. Again, the child's ability to do this is often limited. As noted earlier, the school may have a dress code that forbids wearing the type of clothing which might best conceal the condition. Concealment may also be closed to children whose parents believe it is either a sin or "socially incorrect" for children (especially boys) to wear make-up. In addition, while adults are free to select and purchase their own clothing with the object of concealment in mind, children's clothes are often purchased *for them* by their parents.

Similarly, the custom of parents accepting invitations to social gatherings on behalf of their children results in the children's inability to avoid situations which reveal their stigma.

Other Social Factors

Of course, there are other such variables which may enhance or diminish the impact of impaired appearance of children.

Social class, as mentioned in Chapter Two, is one such factor. Wealthy parents can afford to: (1) receive good prenatal care, thus reducing chances of bearing disfigured children; (2) live in safer environments in terms of both crime and accidents; (3) have their children monitored more closely to avoid accidents; (4) take advantage of the best medical and surgical care, should a child become disfigured; (5) use various concealment strategies; and (6) if need be, provide psychological care for children who are worried about appearance. Finally, in the worst scenario, the wealthy can permit the child to withdraw totally from the outer society, through the employment of tutors, governesses, and other "helpers."

Race is another important consideration. Because our society discriminates against racial minorities, the appearance-impaired child of color may be doubly stigmatized (if poor, triply, and quadruply, if also female). A depigmenting problem such as vitiligo is much more visible on dark skin. Further, a number of ethnic groups have beliefs that contribute to the child's victimization. For example, there is a belief in East Indian culture that any depigmentation is a harbinger of leprosy. During our work with vitiligo patients, Dr. Porter and I learned that some Black Americans believe that vitiligo is God's retributive justice on those who have secretly wished themselves white. Several patients who became totally depigmented were rejected by their communities and their families.

Given all these considerations, it should be clear that being an appearance-impaired child in America will be at best a difficult experience, and sometimes even a tragic one. Our individualistic and materialistic value system with its low tolerance for ugliness, a widespread and universal concept of Anglo-Saxon beauty and cultural ambivalence about children, and a fairly low level of institutional support for appearance-impaired children, combine to produce a situation of considerable difficulty for such children.

Chapter 4

"Funny Looking Kids": Social Stigmatization and Objectification of Appearance-Impaired Children

> Fat persons are related to in (devalued) categorical terms and their self-conceptions may be shaped accordingly. There is a tendency, furthermore, to hold fat persons responsible for their condition—at least implicitly. Fatness is not viewed simply as a physical state, but also evidence of some basic character defect.
>
> Edwin M. Schur
> *Labeling Women Deviant*, 66–72

Sources of Stigmatization

In all the situations in which I have worked, either the appearance-impaired children or their parents report some form of socially stigmatizing incidents. For purposes of discussion, the sources of the stigmatization can be grouped into four categories: (1) total strangers; (2) acquaintances and peers; (3) close friends and family members; and (4) professionals (primarily doctors and teachers).

STRANGERS

"Total strangers" are people unknown to the child. They are mostly encountered in public places, but sometimes also in social gatherings or even in one's own home. The second group will normally not remain strangers, but move into the "acquaintance" category after introductions have been made. Nonetheless, we must treat the first interaction of the child with such people as one of child/total stranger rather than child/acquaintance. Another difference between the two types of strangers is that total strangers who will not become acquaintances are freed from many social norms of the sort that govern social exchanges between people who know one another. Total strangers of this type (the "street" type) may ask rude questions, mock the child, or engage in avoidance behavior, actions prohibited to the stranger destined to become an acquaintance. It is no wonder that total strangers are the group about which children complain the most. The following case brings out many of the characteristics of the encounter between children with impaired appearance and total strangers.

June, a pre-adolescent white female, recalls an incident in the restaurant of a posh department store. Several years before, her mother had instituted a tradition of taking her daughter to the store to see the Christmas decorations and to have lunch. It was a very special event for the child and she looked forward to it eagerly every year. June has a slight patch of vitiligo on her face.

On the special day when she was twelve, she and her mother became aware of two women at a nearby table who were staring at June. They continued to stare, and one of them shook her head, while clicking her tongue in pitying fashion. This continued for some time until the mother became irritated and spoke to the pair. "Is there something I can do for you?" she asked.

"Oh my," replied the clucking woman, "What happened to your little girl? Was she burned?"

The mother bravely undertook an explanation of the pigment loss of vitiligo. She explained that it was not contagious, but the woman paid little attention to her, continuing to stare at June.

"Oh she would be pretty if she didn't have *that*," sighed one.

June and her mother left as soon as they were able to flag a waitress and pay the bill. The child was in tears. These strangers had hurt her feelings. They also put an end to a family tradition, as June has refused to enter the store or the restaurant since this event occurred.

In this example we see people engaging in behavior which they would "normally" consider quite rude, and which they would not employ toward someone they knew. The anonymity conferred by "strangerness" frees them from basic courtesy norms.

In this case as in others, we met alone with the mother (as well as with the child). Her response is a rather common one. It is an educative response, which rests on the notion that cruelty and meanness are the results of ignorance and can be exorcised by knowledge. Unfortunately, this is not always the case. The information supplies may even give bullies new material with which to assail the impaired child.

Another child tells us:

Two people was staring at me at the bus stop, and one of them asked me was I burned. The one guy asked did my hands hurt. I told him only an ignorant person would ask. I told him my mom took a bad medicine when she was pregnant and I was born like this. They laughed. I am having lots operations to fix my hands.

(White male of 10 with fin-like hands)

Stigmatization by strangers may be non-verbal. Many children reported fixed stares or glares on the part of strangers, both adults and other children. These people seemed to project certain emotions in their staring, even though they did not speak. Some appeared to be just "curious," while others seemed to be disgusted or repelled. What matters about these non-verbal forms of stigmatization is that they have an impact on the children. The fact that the children tell us about these incidents reveals that the incidents made an impression on them. In addition, children frequently stated that they "felt bad" or were embarrassed by the event.

All groups of children noted the pointing of fingers as a form of non-verbal stigmatization incident. Indeed this form of behavior seems to upset them very much, much more than plain staring or asking rude questions. This may be due to the fact that pointing is a form of behavior which Americans discourage in the earliest socialization periods: "Don't point, dear, just tell us in words, dearie." "Don't do that. It's RUDE to point." Thus to see someone pointing at us is alarming; it implies that there is something so wrong with us that a person is violating a social prohibition because of us.

Finger pointing in our society is also used to declare and attribute blame. To "point the finger" is to accuse. Thus, a person at whom a finger is pointed is in a sense being accused of something—in this case of ugliness.

Some non-verbal ways of stigmatizing deserve special note because they involve what we might call a "pantomime stigma statement," intended to transmit a special stigmatizing message. One example of non-verbal behavior is the overt cleansing or sterilizing of objects, particularly eating utensils and dishes, after their use by an appearance-impaired child, which an adult person reported.

Questions from strangers may be serious, proceeding from curiosity; at other times, they are simply rude or mocking and intended to hurt the victim, such as "When are you going to take off the mask?" These latter questions really should be classified with jeers and taunts rather than questions.

Avoidance behavior is another form of stigmatizing. Overweight children report that if they go into a meeting room or a theater early, people come in later and take all the seats except the ones beside the child with impaired appearance.

Children are extremely aware of and sensitive to stigmatizing incidents. Staring, laughing, the conspiratorial exchange of glances between two strangers, questions both innocent and rude, taunting, name calling and insults, even physical abuse occur. Every child with impaired appearance has experienced at least one of these. Some may only know the stares, others have to struggle to answer queries such as "How did your face *get* like that, anyhow?" Still others have had their lives made truly horrendous by taunting, jeering classmates whose cruelty seems limitless. These observations are consistent with MacGregor's on children needing plastic surgery.[1]

Carrie has been the victim of this severe stigmatization. She is a white child of six, from a working class family in a large Northeastern city. She has spots of depigmented skin on her legs and thighs (vitiligo). She tells the interviewer that the children at school call her names "like Spot" and "they hit on me all the time." At school, she must stay close to the teacher to protect herself from these experiences.

While Martha, a plump pre-teen, was not subjected to such extreme treatment, this daughter of a New York lawyer told us about two types of incidents which bothered her: the teasing remarks of family members and the wolf whistles of Manhattan construction workers.

No one ever actually *said* anything to Rick, a ten-year-old with severe myopia and thick eyeglasses, but he was aware of how everyone stared at him during the first week of the school year and mortified by the fact that in "choosing up" teams for sports, he was always the last selected. In his working class, Catholic school, sports were of great importance, so this treatment really hurt.

Adults who were appearance-impaired as children recall such incidents clearly. Several adults are quoted by Dr. Kenneth Salyer: one adult woman says, "I considered myself a freak for many years. Kids made fun of me. I was very withdrawn and it was a very painful thing for me to grow up with. . . . If I had a child like me, I'd realized that self-image is a real concern. I'd do everything I could to help that person build as good a self-image as possible. This is the one area that has been tremendously neglected."[2]

Many of the adult vitiligo patients that Dr. Porter and I interviewed made similar remarks. Indeed, it is from one of these interviews that this book derives its title. "Beauty *is* the beast. It's all you hear about. It's on the telly, in the journals, in the store windows. It's everywhere. It dogs my footsteps so that I can never forget that I'm different—that I'll never be beautiful."

Adult women in particular engage in pitying behavior which upsets the child. The head shaking and clucking in the restaurant example above are typical of this phenomenon. Several of the myopic children gave examples of total strangers telling them how good-looking they would be if they didn't have to wear glasses. Some of them actually cry and make such remarks as, "Poor child"; "What a shame"; "Isn't that awful."

Although it is not common, there are several instances in which the stigmatizing party went beyond the realm of verbal offense, actually touching the child, as is evident in a story told by a fat child.

> Waiting at the train station after school, she decided to purchase a candy bar from a vending machine. Just as she was making her selection, a woman she had never seen before grabbed her and dragged her away from the machine, saying, "You don't need that. You're fat enough already."

In extreme cases, the appearance-impaired have found their lives in peril. In the Third Reich, the "final solution" was applied to people with visible physical imperfections as well as to Jews and gypsies.[3] Even in our own culture, there are stories of medical personnel letting "monster" babies die.

In a shattering documentary film, a woman severely crippled since birth by cerebral palsy, very intelligent and now a practicing clinical psychologist, talks about her life. During her childhood, the family home caught fire and she was severely burned. The physician in charge sidled up to her parents and said, "I guess you'd just as soon we not save her," implying that a cerebral palsy child isn't worth the massive effort necessary to save her life. Fortunately, the parents did, indeed, want her saved and fought to see that their child was given the best care available.[4]

ACQUAINTANCES AND PEERS

Name calling and ridicule are the stigmatizing weapons of peers. Fred was a handsome child except for large, protruding ears. He later had his ears "fixed" by a pediatric surgeon. His parents, both school teachers, believed that it was essential that the boy undergo this procedure, as they were aware that he was teased unmercifully at school. The other children called him names, such as "dumbo ears" and "Alfred E. Newman." His homeroom teacher didn't see any harm in this and told him to "laugh with them."

Peers in school or at camp may ask questions and tease the child, but most children say that as time passes and they get to know others and become known in the school or community, this kind of behavior becomes less common.

Unfortunately, family members and professionals are not exempt from the tormenter's role. Teachers may tease the child or give the child a nickname related to his or her impaired appearance. They may initiate or enforce rules that make it difficult for the child to conceal the impairment.

Babbi, 11, is a white girl from a lower middle class Irish-American family. Her parents are first generation Americans, and the family is strongly Catholic and ethnically oriented. Her eye was injured when she was only three by a child in the neighborhood who poked her with a stick. She wears hard lenses and glasses. She was going to be fitted for soft lenses when I first met her, and we saw a great change in her following six months of soft lenses.

Prior to receiving lenses, she was very self-conscious about her "ugly" glasses. Just to add to her problems, the temporary use of hard lenses was a disaster. The hard lenses irritated her eyes and she could not do her school work. She also developed an unfortunate habit of pulling at the edge of her eye, a gesture guaranteed to pop the lens out of the eye. Class would then come to a halt, while the teacher and students crawled about, looking for it.

Babbi's mother told us that one of her teachers tried humiliation as a device to "teach" Babbi not to lose the lenses. This teacher complained out loud when she had to re-insert the lens, drawing the jeering attention of the other students to the situation. All of her classmates teased her about this. "She felt like a freak," says her mother.

School wasn't the only place Babbi lost lenses. One was found in the mouth of a babysitter after falling into a bowl of corn flakes.

The story above of the girl with cerebral palsy who was burned illustrates the contemptuous attitude many physicians have toward children with impaired appearance. When a child is born with impaired appearance, many hospital staff members employ the term F.L.K. ("funny-looking kid") to describe the infant to one another.

FAMILY AND CLOSE FRIENDS

Close friends may make comments or display horror. One mother writes (concerning her baby with cleft lip and palate):

> My mother had been telling everyone that Anne had a problem. One of my friends called to see if she could come over, and I thought she'd been told about it, too. But I guess she hadn't. She brought her little eight-year-old daughter with her. She sort of looked at Anne like GASP! and I never saw her again.[5]

Frances MacGregor's work with plastic surgery patients is in basic agreement with all these observations. Even more upsetting is work done by the Salyers which suggests that mothers themselves may be repelled by the infant's appearance and that this may interfere with bonding, the forging of that essential emotional bond between mother and child. One of the mothers states (about her baby with cleft palate) "I remember in the hospital thinking she has a face that only a mother could love. Then I felt guilty about that."[6]

The Salyers studied behavioral interaction between mothers and craniofacially disfigured newborns in contrast to a group of mothers and "normal" babies. They also administered a questionnaire to the parents regarding their feelings about parenthood. Although the parents of disfigured children differed little from the control parents in self-reported behavior and attitude, actual observation of behavior showed that they:

> held their infants less, touched them affectionately less, and smiled and laughed less. In addition, these mothers provided less tactile-kinesthetic stimulation and vocalization to their infants. In turn, the craniofacially deformed infants smiled less, cried more and averted their heads and bodies more often.[7]

In fact, the authors of *Craniofacial Deformity: A Booklet for Parents* state that facial abnormalities may interfere with initial bonding as well as having long psychological complications:

> The emphasis our society places on physical attractiveness may even influence a mother's ability to bond with her child. These children go on to develop different concepts of friendship, self-worth and self-esteem that influence their entire personality development.[8]

There are two important considerations raised by this research. The first is that even at the very earliest developmental stage, that which Erikson has called "trust versus mistrust," stigmatizing and objectifying may occur that will affect the personality of the child.[9] In fact, we must be very concerned about this because it may interfere with the development of feelings of competency and self-esteem, on which we will place great emphasis in Chapter Five as valuable coping resources.

It has long been recognized that a successful transition through the first year of life characterized by maternal bonding, parental affection, and reliability is necessary for the development of the child's sense of a separate and valued self and for the development of self-esteem. For whatever reason, children whose early days are not characterized by these positive factors may feel rejected and unable to trust the environment, and may have lower confidence and self-esteem.

The Salyers' research also brings to our attention the time and manner in which the impairment of appearance occurs. There is a commonly held belief that children born with impaired appearance are somehow better off, less affected by their condition than those afflicted later, presumably because they have never known a different life. This belief sees children who *acquire* disfigurement later in life as more upset because they can remember their former, more attractive selves. This research suggests quite the opposite—that the child born unimpaired is treated to a normal bonded relationship with parents which will provide the basis for strong psychological coping resources to be used at a later date, while the child impaired at birth may never have the kind of environment needed to produce such resources.

The fact of impairment at birth also suggests the possibility of guilty and angry feelings of parents toward themselves and their spouses in the effort to place blame for the disorder. The acquisition by the child of the disorder through accident or injury will likely not involve these feelings unless the parent actually played a role in the matter, such as abusing the child, or driving a car in an accident in which the child was disfigured. Guilt is a complex feeling and may manifest itself in many ways detrimental to the child, as when a parent projects his or her own sense of guilt onto the child, or withdraws from interacting with the child because of such feelings.

PHYSICIANS

In Chapter Two, I noted that stigmatizing incidents often are also occasions of social objectification. That is, by focusing on the master-status of "person-with-impaired-appearance" and thus ignoring the traits possessed by the child as an individual, the stigmatizer manages to reduce the victim to the position of a *thing* rather than a *person*.

Use of the "F.L.K." term constitutes an act of objectification. So does any use of language that refers to the child by his or her disorder such as "the cleft palate in room 320."

Many children with impaired appearance have had negative experiences with physicians. Many times the first doctor they saw was a non-specialist—a general practitioner or pediatrician who had little or no knowledge about the condition. Many parents felt that these doctors had failed to treat or refer the children adequately.

There was also a frequent complaint that doctors tended to trivialize appearance-related disorders as "only cosmetic." The mothers of vitiligo patients and of anorexics told of taking their children to the doctor as soon as they noted the symptoms of the condition. In many cases, they were told to ignore it; in others, the doctor knew what was wrong but asserted that there was no way to treat it. Children who eventually wound up in an appropriate treatment center often had come there by unorthodox means, such as hearing about the vitiligo clinic on a late-night talk show, rather than by referral.

Many obese children were told that their "baby fat" would eventually disappear, or "melt off," to use the current jargon. And, as long as their thick glasses functioned, myopic children found their concerns curtly dismissed.

Eddie, an eleven-year-old white boy, has the skin disorder, vitiligo, on his right hand, knees, back and feet. He had the disorder for five years before coming to the clinic. He received no help because the pediatrician said he would outgrow it.

Susie is a sixteen-year-old white female, the adopted child of wealthy midwesterners. She has vitiligo on one leg and on her back; it is not [in street clothes] visible. At the onset of the spots, the mother took her to a dermatologist in her own city. He correctly diagnosed it, but would not treat it and told the girl and her family to just ignore it. The mother says that in spite of his cavalier attitude as far as treatment was concerned, "He made it sound catastrophic." The mother then sought advice from her father-in-law who is a doctor, who knew of an East Coast clinic, and the family flew east to seek help. They were pleased with the treatment and have kept it up, flying to the clinic several times a year.

Trivialization was used by many doctors to remind the children of people who were worse off than they were: "You're lucky you aren't blind." "You're lucky you don't have cancer." "You're lucky you aren't diabetic."

The reasons for such treatment are complex. Surely doctors do not set out to wound the feelings of their young patients. Rather, historical, social, and organizational factors combine to create such negative encounters.

First, as medical sociologists have observed, Western medicine has lost its awareness of the inseparable nature of *soma* and *psyche*. While ancient Greek medicine stressed the unity of mind and body and recognized the importance of psychological well-being in the healing process, the Middle Ages witnessed the philosophical separation of the two. The body was delegated to barbers and university-trained physicians; the mind or "spirit" was delegated to the Church. Despite various social movements stressing homeopathic medicine, the notion of the duality of mind and body lingers on, and can still be seen in many medical settings. The major change that has occurred is that in our rather secular society, the mind has been delegated to a new set of specialists, psychiatrists.

American medical education falls short in teaching future physicians to be concerned about patients' states of mind. Nor does it offer training in the communication skills needed to address emotional issues, instead stressing only scientific and technological matters. This makes it difficult to deal with the concerns of appearance-impaired children when they arise.

In addition, specialization has proceeded to such a point that the doctor dealing with a child with impaired appearance does not normally know the child or the family well. The doctor resolves this situation all too often by concentrating totally on the illness, rather than considering the total child.

Linked to both the above tendencies is the custom of doctors of avoiding uncomfortable topics by referring them to psychiatrists rather than attempting to deal with them themselves.

Doctors have been taught in medical schools to judge the serious-ness of a medical problem in terms of its life-threatening nature. By this standard, cosmetic disorders are automatically deemed insignifi-cant. Yet from a child's perspective such problems may seem over-whelming.

Finally, the "corporate invasion of medicine," which is in the pro-cess of transforming health care delivery systems into profit-making enterprises, makes demands on doctors to be fast and efficient, to see *more* patients each day to improve profitability, not spend time an-swering patients' questions or addressing their concerns.

Some of these for-profit organizations actually monitor the amount of time that doctors spend with patients. Those who spend "too much time" with their patients are reminded that this behavior is frowned upon, because it is not bringing in more income. A few organizations use such a monitor to determine reappointments and salaries.

The attribution to a child with impaired appearance of other re-lated characteristics is also objectifying, as we saw in Chapter Two. I have often heard people, with an authoritative tone, hold forth on the personality traits of overweight children. If a child is chubby, these people just *know* that he or she is sulky, spoiled, impatient, and a show-off. Similarly, myopic children wearing thick glasses are thought to be serious, studious "nerds." Yet wearing contact lenses these same children may be regarded as outgoing.

VULNERABILITY TO STIGMATIZATION

The likelihood of a child's being the butt of stigmatizing and objectifying experiences can be thought of in terms of the model set forth in Chapter Two. The child is more or less vulnerable according to his or her situation with regard to:

1. The society's socio-cultural ambiance
2. Visibility, severity, and permanence of the stigma
3. Developmental age

4. Social resources
5. Personality resources
6. The level of social interaction at which the action takes place

The little girl who told of being "hit" by peers, for example, is highly vulnerable in many of these regards.

1. First, as Chapter Three indicated, American society is harsh with respect both to being a child and to being appearance-impaired.
2. This child's stigma is highly visible, severe, and not likely to be repaired.
3. At the age of six and in first grade, she is still not well known to her peers, who may in fact express their own feelings of newness and uncertainty by bullying others.
4. She is from a poor, uneducated family, without much influence in the community.
5. Personality resources are not impressive. The girl is not a happy, "fun," or kind child, and has no great enthusiasm for art, music, or sports.
6. Most of her problems occur at the third level: community, where her resources are weak, but her siblings also do not help her. Neither the wider circle of the school nor the center core of the family act to support her.

A more positive example is that of Robert, whose ethnic ties and strong family support have helped him respond to stigmatization. Robert is an Italian-American of ten, whose vision was impaired in a sports accident two years ago. He is from a solid blue collar family who still reside in the same part of the city as did his parents, grandparents, and great grandparents. The family are very involved in church and community.

Robert says he will wear glasses, "just for sometime" as he looks "ugly" in them. On the other hand, he has had trouble with hard contact lenses because he keeps losing them.

Robert's situation is interesting in terms of Goffman's notion of the "discredited" and the "discreditable."[10] A person in a social situation can be referred to as "discreditable" if the stigmatizing characteristic is not known and cannot be seen. He or she is "discredited" either if the impairment or other deviance is immediately obvious, or if it *becomes* apparent. Robert with glasses is one of the discredited. Contact lenses offer him the opportunity to hide his myopia and to engage in activities, especially sports activities. The disguise is a faulty one, however, because the lenses fall out and become lost. The ensuing search makes him the center of unwanted attention, and he again becomes discredited. Wryly, he told me of a trip to the ball park to watch the Phillies that ended up with "the Phillies and everyone else watching me," as he, his family, and helpful strangers crawled around the stands looking for it.

Robert's mother attends to the care of his lenses, but his father does not encourage special treatment of his son. Rather, he has encouraged Robert to accept his condition and take a "business as usual" attitude.

Robert is a good-natured child and quite outgoing. He does well at school, and is active in a tight ethnic community. Looking at Robert we can immediately see that, despite a lack of wealth or personal skills, the support that the family gives him, and in turn the family's secure status within the Italian community, are strong. He can also feel good about the repairability of his affliction, which in time will make him "normal."

Susie also presents a positive picture. At sixteen she has vitiligo on the leg and back, which is not visible when she is dressed. Susie's mother says she is dealing with this problem, "very well" now, better than when she was younger. She does worry about summer and the beach, because the areas of her body with vitiligo are more visible in a bathing suit, and because the white areas stand out more as her normal skin tans.

Susie also says that the condition bothered her a lot at first, but less now. People do stare and make remarks, but she feels that is "their problem." If people ask what the white spots are, in a non-insulting way, she gives them an educational response. She tells us that her family have been very supportive, as has her boyfriend.

Susie is attractive and well-spoken, and has a good sense of humor. She has a clearly defined goal—to become a veterinarian.

Susie's case thus indicates a situation of a very positive sort:

1. The disorder is only visible under certain circumstances (bathing suit, shorts).
2. It is not widespread.
3. It is being treated with some signs of remission.
4. She has many personal resources: beauty of face, intelligence, a good sense of humor, clear-cut career goals.
5. She also has many social resources: wealth, status in her community, a supportive boyfriend and parents, and connections (through her grandfather) to the clinic.
6. She has passed through the early adolescent obsession with appearance and moved into an older-teen stage with concerns about career decisions and the ability to form close intimate relationships.

Chapter Five demonstrates how these same factors are of importance in determining the child's reaction to stigmatization. That chapter also shows how the model developed in Chapter Two can be used as the basis for a detailed assessment of the "coping status" of appearance-impaired children. Assessments of Robert and Susie are included in that discussion (see Tables 2 and 5).

Chapter 5

Coping with Impaired Appearance

> The foundations of the psychological symptoms often found in older (cranial-facial) patients begin very early in life. The emphasis our society places on physical attractiveness may even influence a mother's ability to bond with her child. These children go on to develop different concepts of friendship, self-worth, and self-esteem that influence their entire personality development.
>
> *Craniofacial Deformity; A Booklet for Parents,* pp. 2–3

Acts of stigmatization produce a wide variety of responses. Some children seem quite impervious to them, while others are badly hurt and some may even become self-destructive. The majority attempt to cope as best they can and often manage to overcome the unkindnesses with which they must constantly deal.

This chapter is concerned with what factors help or hinder the coping process.

In Chapter Two, I noted Pearlin's three categories of coping strategies for situations that cause stress.[1] They can be paraphrased for stigmatizing events:

1. Those which attempt to prevent the stigmatizing event from happening by changing the situation around it;
2. those which attempt to change the meaning of the stigmatizing event; and
3. those which attempt to control stress after the stigmatizing event has happened.

Appearance-impaired children employ, or attempt to employ, all these strategies, but generally must rely on those in category 3— *coping* in various ways with the stigmatizing events in their world.

Preventing or Changing the Meaning of Stigmatizing Events

Some children attempt to hide their stigmatizing condition as a way of preventing the recurrence of stigmatizing events, Pearlin's first approach. This strategy recalls Goffman's distinction between "discredited" and "discreditable."[2] Goffman's concentration on this distinction derives in part from the fact that he was dealing with various sorts of stigma. A "bad habit," for example, like alcoholism or drug addiction, is a stigma not at once or always visible to others. A person can save face by engaging in it only while totally alone where no one can witness and label the behavior, and thus not be discredited. In the case of odd-looking children, we are mainly dealing with people who *are* discredited. Being odd-looking cannot be hidden very easily. Even if attempts are made to do so, they are usually unsuccessful, or, the attempts themselves may be so odd as to be somewhat bizarre in their own right. Too much make-up, long gloves in the summer, high scarves, or dark glasses may attract the very attention that the wearer sought to avoid.

There are *degrees* of discreditation, however, which rest mainly on the visibility of the impairment. In this respect, we must acknowledge that Mary, who has pale, white splotches on ebony skin but whose disfigurement is limited to the legs, is not so obviously impaired as John, an Asian-American child with less pronounced spots on his face. From a social perspective, the face is by far the most critical of body parts.[3] And it is almost impossible to hide facial impairment. The child with marred legs or arms is able, albeit in a limited fashion, to camouflage or cover up the disorder. However, as we shall see later in the discussion, this effort is rarely totally successful, and is an anxiety-producing strategy for the child, who constantly fears the discovery of the problem by others, and it often means passing up pleasant experiences and social opportunities if they are associated with possible revelation of the impairment. Many of the children with vitiligo on their legs or torsos seek to avoid outdoor summer activities, especially at a beach or pool. They may also attempt to avoid school regulations, such as communal showers after gym, which would reveal their depigmentation to the other children.

Children also employ the second strategy, seeking to *change the meaning of the stigmatizing event*. For example, several parents told us that their children pretended not to hear remarks shouted at them on the street.

One anorexic patient told me that, during the "fat phase" prior to her dramatic weight loss, construction workers would shout "fat" remarks at her, but she would tell herself and others that the workers were shouting sexual remarks of a complimentary nature.

Most children have to take Pearlin's third approach and *cope with the stress of stigma* when it occurs. Some of them do this well, while others find it difficult.

Saving Face

"Saving face," a phrase commonly used to indicate the retention of one's dignity, takes on an ironic aspect when applied to the efforts of appearance-impaired children to maintain their dignity, for often one's face has been the source of that which threatens one's dignity and self respect. As we have seen, children with impaired appearance of all sorts are universally exposed to embarrassing incidents, focusing on their impairment. Although, as we have seen already and will discuss in more detail in the next sections, such factors as visibility, social class, and age do cause some differences, all experience some embarrassment and psychological stress caused by the stares, questions, rude remarks, and jeers described above.

The issue we address in this chapter is what impact such treatment has on the child. Is the child able to deal effectively with these incidents and maintain good humor and self respect? Or is the child

TABLE 1
Assessment

U. S. Culture	Social Resources
	Parental support
Age	Parental attitude
	Parents' education
Competency	Wealth
	Prestige/honor
Physiological Resources	Community/school involvement
Visibility	Family stability
Severity	(Total)
Repairability	
	Levels of Interaction
Psychological Resources	Core—family, friends
Humor	Neighbors, acquaintances
Creativity	Larger community
Intelligence	Unknown
Friendliness	(Total)
Self-esteem	
	Total

negatively influenced by such events, becoming shy, embittered, withdrawn, angry, or self-effacing because of this treatment. Can the children, in at least some instances, become the victims of self-stigmatization, accepting a self-definition totally rooted in and determined by society's negative view and its arm's-length reaction to their appearance? Such variations in responses of the victims of impaired appearance are not random, but are related to physiological, sociological, and psychological variables.

The children's interviews themselves suggested four levels of response to impaired appearance: (1) The child reported some negative incidents associated with it, but was only mildly concerned with the disorder and seemed well adjusted. (2) The child was moderately concerned with the impaired appearance, and worried but was not depressed, withdrawn, or preoccupied with it. (3) The child was very concerned about the appearance impairment and expressed this con-

TABLE 2
Assessment: Susie

U. S. Culture	−	Social Resources	
		Parental support	+
Age	+	Parental attitude	+
		Parents' education	+
Competency	+	Wealth	+
		Prestige/honor	+
Physiological Resources		Community/school involvement	+
Visibility	+	Family stability	+
Severity	+	(Total)	(7)
Repairability	+		
		Levels of Interaction	
Psychological Resources		Core—family, friends	+
Humor	+	Neighbors, acquaintances	+
Creativity	−	Larger community	−
Intelligence	+	Unknown	−
Friendliness	+	(Total)	(2)
Self-esteem	+		
		Total	18

cern through preoccupation, depression, or withdrawal. (4) The child was very concerned and expressed it through hostility, anger, and denial.

This chapter works with the interviews with appearance-impaired children and their parents collected in the various studies described earlier in this volume, to identify and characterize these relationships in terms of the model developed in Chapter Two (and shown in Figure 1). A child's "coping status" can be assessed in terms of the factors in the model. The assessment can then be presented in table form as a help to professionals, family, and others involved in helping the child. Table 1 shows a blank assessment chart. Table 2 is a chart completed for "Susie," the myopic child described in Chapter Four.

The categories used in these tables derive from the model and discussion in earlier chapters, and are described in more detail in the next few sections of this chapter. In the assessment process, the various factors are identified as + or − depending on whether they are working favorably or unfavorably for the child.

Age

The description above should make clear that none of these factors acts in isolation. It is impossible to discuss even such a "quantifiable" parameter as age without dealing as well with family support and other elements. The children are of many ages; we can impose some order on the data by examining children in different developmental age groups as to how successfully they are coping with impaired appearance.

The children fall into the groups and age-specific concerns shown in Table 3. Not all children of a given age will follow the trends noted here, and many will combine more than one age pattern.

The lines between these categories are also blurred. A sixteen-year-old may still be fixated on looks, while a ten-year-old may not have entered the period of concern with appearance and conformity.

Of course we must remember that to some extent what importance age will have on a child will depend on other factors. One can be at a "bad age"—such as the pre-teen, early adolescent concern with beauty—and yet do well because of a supportive family, good friends, and a good sense of humor.

On the other hand, for someone like the Elephant Man, ugliness was and remained a "master status," no matter what age he was; so we must take severity into account in weighing our evidence for the importance of developmental age.

Yet there is little research on the importance of age (or developmental stage) on the child's ability to cope with impaired appearance. We know the pre-school years to be devoted to the acquisition of ego skills.[4] Here, impaired appearance could contribute to strained interaction with the primary group.

During the elementary school years, the central developmental task confronting the child is the mastering of the technology of his or

TABLE 3
Age-Specific Developmental Concerns

AGE	DEVELOPMENTAL CONCERN	EFFECT FOR APPEARANCE-IMPAIRED
0–18 mo.	Building a sense of self separate from mother's body. Ability to trust, to be sure of mother's love.	If loved, if trust built now, will be a vital strength through life.
18 mo.–5	Learning to talk, walk, go one's own way. Independence and autonomy acquired.	If parent over-rules, child has no faith in self. Permissiveness also a danger. Child fears lack of parameters.
6–9	Learning to take initiative-to plan something and carry it through to completion. At school industriousness and the economic skills of society.	Very important in self esteem. Parents doing it for child prevent child from mastering skills.
9–15	Superficial appearance, being accepted, being a member of a group.	Overlaps with junior-high years. A hard time for appearance-impaired.
16–20	Finding a loved companion and security in a relationship with this person. Deciding on life's work.	Can be a good time, if not too scarred by earlier experiences. Love and work ethos obscures earlier emphasis on superficial appearance.

her society—be it bow and arrow or complicated reading and mathematical skills. It is a time of learning, of gaining a sense of the competence of one's self. Any factor that prevents this sense of master threatens the psychological well-being of the child at this stage in the life cycle.

In addition, the importance of mastering one's body—also an important aspect of this stage of development—is being learned through sports, dance, and other physical activity. Competency could, as stated above, help the child. However, bad experiences at school related to appearance could slow the acquisition of competency feelings.

Appearance becomes an important aspect of one's sense of self in the early teens.[5] This is true of children of both sexes, but is especially important for girls. Being like others, belonging to the group, feeling accepted as a person, are all key factors for the young person of this age.[6] Feelings of well-being have been linked to the degree of happiness experienced in terms of satisfaction with appearance during adolescence;[7] these feelings and the confidence they bring with them may carry over well into the adult years.

A consideration of these stages suggests that the early adolescent, especially the younger adolescent (9–13), for whom body image is of great importance, is the most embarrassed by impaired appearance. Younger children are occupied with other concerns, and later adolescents have to concern themselves with more demanding issues: whether to attend college, what career or occupation to pursue, the selection of a mate. Thus, we might expect extreme concern with appearance to diminish as we move into the older teens.

Dawn is a twelve-year-old white girl whose eyes were injured in a car accident several years ago. Although surgery helped to repair her vision, she must wear one hard lens and glasses. At the time of our interview, she was hoping to graduate to soft lenses in both eyes, but it was uncertain whether this would be a realizable goal.

She is consumed by the importance of appearance, a tendency not unusual in girls of her age.

She is still unable to put in or remove the lens herself. Her mother does this as well as the cleaning and sterilization of the lens.*

*Dawn's goal of soft lenses was in fact realized. See Table 6 below. It is interesting to note that, in my sample of myopic children using contact lenses, all had assumed care for their own lenses except the three whose vision problem was the result of trauma. Although they all fell into pre-teen age groups, they continued this dependency, while younger children took care of their own lenses.

Dawn is a moderate coper. If we apply the model to her case, we can see that while family support is present, it is rather muted. In talking with the mother, one certainly feels the love and concern she has for her child, but there is a tension here. There is also guilt about the circumstances under which the eyes were damaged. It was unclear to me whether the mother was a passenger in the car or the driver; in any case, there is much remorse and the mother repeatedly shakes her head and talks about how pretty the child "used to be."

Actually, Dawn is a very pretty child, well dressed, with green eyes and blond hair. She wants to get rid of her glasses. In fact she often removes them in order to look "better." Dawn feels that she looks very ugly when wearing glasses. Her friends contribute to these feelings, telling her repeatedly how much prettier she is without her glasses.

Dawn says that she is anxious about entering a room full of "new" people because she feels that they are all looking at her glasses. In fact, when she knows a "special" social occasion is important to her, she contrives to leave her glasses at home. The opinions that others have of her are very important for her as they are for any pre-teen, but the need for acceptance is enhanced by the embarrassment of wearing spectacles.

In a separate interview with Dawn's mother, we learn that this concern with appearance has increased over the past two years. Dawn seemed relatively unconcerned about it at 7 or 8 years of age.

Dawn has few interests and is doing poorly in school. She likes swimming, but the school will not let her swim competitively with contact lenses, and she can't see well enough to compete without them.

M.B. is a sulky white male of thirteen from a high-paid blue collar home. He seemed hostile to the interviewer, and manifested this by answering "Who knows?" to every question she asked. He developed the white spots of vitiligo on the area of his left hand where he had been injured in a bike accident. It spread all over the hand.

M.B. is also a denier. He tells us he has no worries and doesn't have any bad experiences. He has quit the clinic.

The only positive response we were able to generate was about his home. He is very proud of his home, which is out in the country and has a pool for swimming and ice skating. He also likes to draw and paint his home.

After the strenuous effort needed to elicit any responses from the child, the mother came as a pleasant surprise. She is very friendly and outgoing. She states that her son seemed unbothered by his condition until sixth grade. At that time they moved and he had to go to a new school and deal with new people. This all took place around the time of her remarriage.

This child struck me as very angry. He was hostile to the interviewer, to the medical staff, and to his mother during the time they were in the waiting room.

Overall, this is an unhappy case, except for the happiness with the new house. He is in the most vulnerable age group, he seems to have no important psychological resources, the mother is supportive, but "a new father" is always a source of stress, under the best of circumstances.

Reviewing the case we can see that this child has experienced three major transitions recently: the loss of his real father (by death or divorce), changing residence, and going to a new school—quite a lot to handle, especially with a visible disorder, and during the developmental stage when being accepted is of crucial importance.

Thus it would appear that transition or changes exacerbate the tendency of certain age groups to become depressed or anxious.

The age 0–18 months was discussed when we examined the feelings of parents of infants born with impaired appearance. We noted that these parents may be less responsive to their infants and may even fail to bond with them. As this is the critical stage for the development of self-esteem, anything which threatens bonding or the parents' quick response to the infant's expression of need may impair the development of self-esteem, which is also an important psychological resource later in life.

During the next two stages (5–12 years, i.e., the elementary school years) independence and learning in school are important.

The relationship between the autonomy/independence factor and response to stigma is complex, for it is also apparent that children whose sense of autonomy has been nurtured prior to, or in spite of, disfigurement, pay less attention to appearance in general because they are more likely to be involved in fascinating activities. A good example of this is Bobbie, a four-year-old black child with very visible spots of depigmentation on his face. Bobbie is little concerned with appearance at this point in his life, however, because he is on a "learning roll," as I came to call it. The child is virtually in love with learning, and his curiosity and desire to practice what he has learned are actively encouraged by loving parents. (It is interesting to accentuate the plural of parents here. Bobbie's father, a serious, gentle person, is very involved, and records show that he frequently accompanies his wife and son to the vitiligo clinic.)

Venturing a bit far afield from Freud's rigid adherence to the notion that all developmental stages hinge only on the resolution of conflict centered around erogenous zones, we can link this period in the child's personality formulation to the newly developed ability to play a decisive role in his or her own actions. This ability is related to physiological and cultural factors.

The child gains what we might call "the power of negativity" during the second year in two major acquisitions: (1) the ability to walk, trot, and eventually to gallop at a fairly impressive clip; (2) and the ability to speak and thus negate.

"Come here, Billy," calls mother. Billy gives her a big smile and runs like crazy in the opposite direction.

"OK, Wendy, let's go wash our hands before lunch!" says the day-care worker. "No." responds Wendy though not necessarily unamiably.

Negativity is tied closely to the young child's quest for the independence and autonomy so necessary for developing a separate and positive sense of self. In the years between two and six, children test the limits of their new autonomy through the invocation of negativity. Anyone who has spent any time in the presence of the "terrible twos" knows that "no" is the most popular word in the child's vocabulary.

The successful resolution of this stage rests on the ability of mature parents to remain unthreatened by the many challenges to their authority, and to give the child enough choices and enough occasions successfully to assert his or her own wishes (without becoming a small tyrant who rules the family by tantrums, while really trembling inwardly at the power of his or her own unlimited passion and willfulness). A child without limits is a child afraid.

In the life-long process of building ego strength or self-esteem, this stage is of considerable importance because the concept of autonomy involves the ability of an individual to act on his or her own, to make independent choices that affect other aspects of life, to be able to stand and act and be alone without feeling lonely or inadequate. It is a good time to accentuate the positive, to recognize the areas in which a child has interests or ability and to cultivate them.

A less autonomous self will emerge in situations where the child's efforts at independence have been misinterpreted by the adults in his or her life as rebellious willfulness and have been punitively extinguished. Bullying parents may score a short-term victory, apparently exacting unquestioning obedience from their children, but a price will have been paid; that price is the confidence of the children in themselves as independent, autonomous actors. They become frightened adults who seek to identify with powerful, dictatorial leaders or rigid, inflexible organizations that continue to play the authoritarian role in their lives that the parents once played. Members of the Nazi party, or the ill-fated followers of the Rev. Jones who led his admirers into mass suicide by poisoning in Guyana, are examples of this outcome.

Unfortunately, some loving and well-meaning parents handle the stage of autonomy almost as ineffectively as harsh ones. Doting parents can overprotect children, permitting them little or no autonomy out of a desire to protect the child from all possible harm or encounters with failure. But feelings of personal efficacy are rooted in failure as well as in success. As Skolnick has observed, *failure,* when it results from one's own actions, testifies to the fact that one has had *some* effect on the environment, whereas success brought about by the overprotectiveness of others does not teach the child that what he or she does may have an impact.[8]

In the situation of children with impaired appearance, the temptation to overprotect is very strong. Parents fear that cruelty on the part of others may hurt their child in some critical, elemental sense. In order to prevent harm to the child from prying questions, mean taunts, ridicule, and shame, parents may limit the child's exposure to new people and new experiences. In the case where disfigurement is limited to a certain part of the body, they may avoid social situations that reveal or highlight that part of the child's anatomy. For example, parents of several of the children with vitiligo on their backs or trunks reported reluctance to permit their children to go to the beach or to swimming pools because the condition was revealed by bathing attire, and also because exposure to the sun makes vitiligo more visible by darkening the normal areas of pigmentation around the very white depigmented areas. A number of young children reported teasing remarks and questions taking place in such settings, but they did not appear nearly so upset about it as their parents. In fact, children of this age learned quite quickly how to deal with such situations *if* they were given repeated opportunity to visit the beach or pool. "I be a teacher!" says Rachel, who followed her mother's counsel that questions and teasing are merely the products of ignorance. "I tell them that some dark cells die and it's not contagious. So forget it."

Parents who become upset and respond by keeping the child away from provocative settings deprive the child of the opportunity to develop coping strategies and they increase the child's sense of dependency on adults.

In addition, the children are rarely unaware of the parents' emotional response. Two adolescents, looking back, remembered near-hysterical responses to vitiligo on the part of their parents. Seventeen-year-old Jenny said "I was at a sleep-over camp in New England. I was six. When my mother came up for Parents' Day and saw me, she just started to cry. I really hadn't paid much attention to those white spots on my legs, but she made a big deal out of it."

The young child (3–6) seems relatively unaffected by appearance impairment, even when the disorder is quite visible. Children of this age are still quite centered on family and self. A loving set of parents can provide a fortress against the hurts which come later as the social worlds expand. These children are able to believe that they are, indeed, beautiful because their parents say they are, despite very visible impairments in appearance. In addition, life holds so many challenges and satisfactions for them that they do not tend to focus much on appearance. A young boy of four with widespread and visible vitiligo exemplified this exuberance for life. This child made friends with everyone in a clinic waiting room, drew many pictures during the period between the interview and his treatment, wrote the entire alphabet several times (each time in a different color of ink), wrote all numbers from 1 to 20 several times, looked at and commented on all of the pictures in the hall, and, in general, was quite engaged with his environment throughout his visit. Another four-year-old with severe facial burn scars confided that she spends most of her "free" time making books. She illustrates and composes the text with some adult help.

This pattern of minor difficulty as a result of appearance impairment seems to continue throughout most of early childhood. There is some evidence in the cases of six-year-olds that the first year of school may be an exception. It involves concern about meeting new people, leaving the protective environment of the home, and having to conform to new sets of norms. Being called names or teased at school causes children much distress. This feeling was pronounced in several of the myopic children who were teased about wearing glasses.

However, this situation seems to abate as the child begins to feel more at ease in school and becomes known by peers.

A more impressive change seems to occur in the pre-pubertal years and in some cases it endures through the early teens. This period (9–13) is marked by anxiety about appearance, a greatly increased amount of time spent thinking about the impairment, efforts at cover-up, profound shyness around new people, and extreme modesty with one's peers. Of course some of these factors are simply a part of normal adolescent development. However, in our patients, anxieties are accentuated because the patients feel they have something to be ashamed of and hide.

Nor does physiological adolescence seem to be the only factor here. According to the children and their parents, the change occurs in anticipation of another transition—the move up to junior high or high school. Anxieties arise about the new location and larger size of the school and the higher level of academic expectations (which seem to heighten the sense of visibility). Concern about dating arrives. Body/beauty concerns triggered by the high school practice of group showering for sports were mentioned by several children. This seems to be the most difficult age for children. In the film "Mask," a severely deformed child has done well in grade school and has many friends, but with adolescence he becomes depressed.

E.V., an eleven-year-old, has vitiligo on his right hand, knees, back and feet. He had this condition for five years before going to the vitiligo clinic. He has been receiving treatment there for one year. His mother, who refers to him as her "gorgeous kid," brought him to the clinic. Both she and the boy say that he was much less concerned about his appearance when he was younger, but his concern has increased, especially during the past year.

There is considerable trouble at home. The mother broke down, during our talk, and told me that her husband has all the difficulties of the Post Viet Nam syndrome, and is suicidal and alcoholic.

She is holding down two jobs and another child has been very ill. She also said that E.V. had been in a car accident the week before while with a paternal uncle. He was drenched with gasoline in the crash and became quite upset, comparing it to his father's experience in Viet Nam.

As stated above, she feels he coped better with the vitiligo as a small child. During the past year, he became quite anxious about it. She observes that this anxiety coincided with his worry of going to junior high school, especially the much discussed common showers following gym classes.

E.V. is a handsome youngster whose skin condition is not visible [in ordinary clothes], except for a small patch on his right hand. He reports incidents of name-calling at the swimming pool, being called "white knees."

He says he ignores such incidents, but it does seem that he is bothered by them.

J.T. is a white male vitiligo patient of thirteen. White spots are obvious on his arms and legs. At the time I interviewed him, there was some remission of vitiligo under a treatment of aspirin and psoralin and exposure to sun light.

J.T. reports that "little kids" have asked him many questions about the disorder. His mother recalls an incident at a grocery store when he was wearing shorts and a girl of his own age questioned him about the "spots."

There have been two recent additions to J.T.'s family: a sister one year old and another aged 2. The interviewer observed the family leaving the clinic; J.T. was holding the two-year-old's hand and carrying the baby. In this role he was very animated and confident and both little girls were beaming at him and smiling.

In this case we see a person of the vulnerable age group (9–13) with a visible appearance impairment, but we do not see the emotional negativity we might expect. What variables can we see here that provide J.T. with a positive outlook? Strong parental support, some remission of the skin disorder, and an important role within the family caring for his sisters.

Older teens, while still somewhat concerned about appearance, seem to derive compensatory satisfaction from the acquiring of skills with which they can later obtain a job, by sports or artistic abilities, and by relationships with their peers.

An interesting example of these trends is to be found in the case of a sixteen-year-old white male with a widespread skin disorder. He has had his impairment since early childhood. Both R and his mother reported little concern about this during the elementary school years. However, in the year prior to going to junior high school and during the junior high school years, R became extremely self-conscious about his appearance, very shy in new social situations and also became quite withdrawn. His parents were very concerned. R had other problems at this time and one suspects that appearance became the lightning rod for a number of these concerns. He was not a good student and when other boys began to mature, he still was a child physically.

At sixteen, however, he was a quite different young man. His disorder was still visible, but he was little concerned with it. In examining his new situation, we find that he has accomplished the early resolution of several psychological tasks. The child and his mother, interviewed separately, both attribute his new adjustment to three factors. The first is his switch to a vocational school where he is learning carpentry. He is very excited about carpentry and looking forward to spending his life at it. Second, at fifteen, his physical maturation took place. He had caught up to other boys in terms of height, weight and secondary sex characteristics. Third, he had a steady girlfriend who "doesn't care" about his disorder and with whom he had a very warm and open relationship.

The age-related changes in emotional response that were noted by the parents as well as the children confirm this pattern. The parents of elementary school children reported no changes; the parents of pre-junior high and junior high school students note a change for the worse, as do the children themselves; and the parents of high school students and the patients themselves note a change for the better.

We have observed that the reactions of children would suggest that the stage of "identity versus role confusion, which Erikson says runs during "adolescence," starts earlier and involves two stages.[9] This does not necessarily mean that Erikson was wrong in establishing the age parameters; instead, we may be witnessing a cultural change in the definition of "early adolescence." This change has been brought about to some degree by the development of "middle schools" and "junior high schools," which define the "pre-" or "early" adolescent as already finished with the stage of industry but not yet fully into adolescence. It is also influenced by the biological fact of earlier menarche in American females (the product of improved nutrition) and the concomitant changes in customs, such as earlier dating.

It would not be worthwhile to belabor this point were it not for the tremendous importance of the early adolescent stage in the lives of children with impaired appearance. Without a doubt, this is the worst time in the life cycle for most patients. Not only can we learn this from retrospective testimony of adults, but the children themselves are much more concerned and socially withdrawn at this time as reported by them and their parents. Around 15 or 16, their concern lessens and they switch to a concern anticipatory of young adulthood—about earning a living and forming intimate relationships. This transformation suggests that the stage of identity versus role confusion may, in fact, have two substages. During the early stage, identity may be an issue of the physical self—an acceptance of pubertal changes and their incorporation into one's body image and an acceptance of one's own physical self as pretty, handsome, socially acceptable to others. The later stage is concerned with what we might call self-in-role, the reaching out to the development of occupational roles, citizen roles, and roles such as lover, spouse, nurturer.

Viewing adolescence in this manner helps us understand the high concern and worry of the ten-to-thirteen-year-old and what seems of lesser concern in the older adolescent.

Of course we must not overlook one very obvious fact. *All* young teens experience some anxiety about their appearance during early adolescence and some of them have poor self-esteem. Thus, in a classic situation of scape-goating, "normal" but anxious young teens, struggling for group acceptance, lash out at the appearance-impaired child to make themselves feel more acceptable. It is, therefore, during this stage of life that our children receive *more stigmatizing experiences* at the hands of their peers. This factor also contributes to this time being the most painful period in the life-cycle for the appearance-impaired.

Competency

Overall, the factor that seems to make the most difference is one which I have called "a feeling of competency." I use this term to denote good self-esteem, but more than that, a child's sense of personal efficacy, a sense that he or she *matters* and is capable of having an impact on the environment. It also implies an awareness that one is "good at" certain things. In studying the reactive coping skills of children with vitiligo, Porter and I found that even children with severe visible vitiligo coped well if they were high in competency feelings.

That study included fascinating cases of children who had severe and highly visible impairment of their faces but were nonetheless doing very well in terms of adjustment and coping. In these cases we find an avid interest in acquiring and using new skills and abilities. They indicate that the satisfaction of ego and competency needs can go a long way in compensating for the degree of impairment in appearance.

This finding is of considerable importance because it suggests the therapeutic power of mastering one's environment. The ego strength of these children is being fortified constantly by the joy that comes from a sense of increased competency.

COMMUNITY RESOURCES

While social class is a fairly moderate force, it does appear that younger working class and poor children encounter more teasing in school and in their neighborhoods. On the other hand, in adolescence, the working class child seemed to have some advantage. Because the working class children planned to work directly after high school, they were already mastering the skills with which they would later earn a living. As noted above, competency feelings mitigate against overconcern with appearance. The middle class child is more likely to be preparing for college and not yet acquiring the actual skills required for a job.

GENDER

There is little difference in coping by gender. Though we might not expect it, boys are as upset about impaired appearance as girls. The notion that appearance is more important to girls has not been confirmed in my experience. But it *is* worth noting that all the very "angry/hostile" responses I have seen are male. This suggests that while members of the two genders are equally disturbed by impaired appearance, this disturbance may be *expressed* differently. Porter and I noted in a discussion of our three *worst* copers:

> As noted above, the pattern of male anger and female depression and withdrawal is typical. The older male patient, a black male of eighteen, is a very recent case and the severity of his reaction may certainly be attributable to that, partly from shock, partly from having had little treatment yet. In addition, it is a bizarre and visible case of unilateral vitiligo. It is as if a line had been drawn down the middle of his face leaving the right side an almost movie-star handsome brown and the left mottled and depigmented. In addition to high visibility, we also note the absence of the father and a lack of interest in school or job or in any activity. Hopefully, treatment, if it is at all successful, will begin to lift his spirits.

The other two cases are white children, ten and thirteen. The girl has vitiligo on her face. Both have experienced recent transitions in their lives. Neither reports an avid interest, skill or hobby. The father of the male patient returned from Vietnam with severe psychological problems. The girl's mother is over-identified with the child and cries frequently at the clinic about the prospect of the girl's future in the marriage market because of impaired appearance. Both situations suggest the absence of very supportive family situations for the children.

Emotional response to impaired appearance in children thus seems to be determined by no one variable, but by the interplay of visibility, feelings of competency, family support, type of treatment program and age.10

In general, it has been my observation that children with a low sense of competency take disfigurement harder and are less likely to devise successful coping strategies than those with high competency feelings. Children low in competency feelings are the most likely to engage in self-stigmatization, accepting the negative view that others have of their impairment.

What goes into creating a sense of competency for children? A combination of factors is involved which include: (1) strong parental love of, and support for, the child; (2) a lack of over-concern with the impairment from the parent or parents and other "significant others," such as siblings, grandparents, and teachers; (3) intelligence; (4) an active interest in *something*—sports, art, music, gymnastics—in which the child invests sincere and concerted energy. It is the involvement in such interests and the effects—diversion of attention outside the self, fascination and joy of learning, the feelings of self-worth that emerge in response to any job well done—which feeds the child's self-esteem and counters society's negative assessment of his or her appearance with pride and self-respect.

Actually, what determines a child's response to disfigurement is the unique combination and patterning in the life of each child of all the factors noted above. This point can be illustrated briefly by the case histories discussed in the following section, which show the interplay of developmental age, visibility, gender, parental attitudes, support of friends, and competency feelings all working together to produce the ability to cope effectively or not.

VISIBILITY AND SEVERITY

The generous response to my requests for data by individuals and organizations concerned with the care of children who suffer from deformities because of such disorders as Sturges-Weber or cleft palate bears strong testimony to the concerns these children also have about the way they look. Yet little is written about these matters, so overshadowed are they, in the eyes of the medical profession, by the other aspects of their disorders.

Our creative artists have been more in the vanguard of drawing attention to the psychological difficulties confronted by such children than have the physicians. Both "The Elephant Man" and "Mask" were movies which demonstrated concern for these matters, as did novelist John Updike's writings on psoriasis.

All too often the medical professional, perhaps ill at ease with emotionally-laden subject matter, sidesteps or even trivializes the issue of appearance. "You're lucky you don't have *lupus*," one teenager was told by her doctor, after confiding in him about her concern for appearance.

Booklets for children with specific disorders are largely devoted to the medical aspects of the problem and may barely touch on the fact that the disorder is extremely disfiguring (that people stare and point, ask questions and make rude remarks), let alone offer advice on how to handle such problems.

It may seem quite obvious that among the determinants of response to disfigurement, the severity and visibility of that disfigurement rank high. What is less obvious, even surprising, is the degree to which they can be mitigated by such non-physical factors as imagination, family support, developmental age, and competency feelings. In addition, a child's response to stigmatization is a product of overall cultural factors such as those we discussed in Chapter Three and may vary according to what level of action we examine.

Examining first the effects of visibility and severity alone, we observe that while increased severity and high visibility frequently co-exist, in situations where they do *not,* visibility is of greater importance in determining response than severity. For example, in the children with vitiligo I studied with Judith Porter, we found that even the presence or absence of a small patch of vitiligo on the face and hands (but especially the face) was more distressful than widespread vitiligo on the torso. Similarly, overweight pre-teens suffer more embarrassment even if they are very moderately chubby than their peers with bulemia, which is a more severe disorder, but not a visible one.

However, new social occasions (transitions) which could lead to the exposure of severe but formally hidden disfigurements are dreaded. A prime example of this is in the dread of group-showering on the part of children who have vitiligo on their torsos but not on such exposed areas as their hands and face. Group showers, a requirement in many high schools, threaten to expose a secret the child has struggled to maintain for perhaps years.

In the importance of visibility, we see an affirmation of the social nature of stigma. If it isn't known and can't be seen, the process of stigmatization *is* unlikely to be set in motion—until and unless the social situation threatens to reveal the stigma. Goffman's terms "discreditable" and "discredited" are applicable here.

One myopic teenager told of her efforts to hide her disorder (before receiving contact lenses) by withholding from boys of her age group the fact that she was extremely nearsighted and needed thick glasses to see adequately. This teenager wore her glasses only in the classroom. As the lesson ended, she would remove her glasses and put them in her book bag.

She did not wear her glasses on dates, and therefore often placed herself in bizarre social situations. For example, she attended many films which she never actually "saw" and had to avoid discussions of these films. She gained a reputation as a snob for her failure to recognize and greet friends in public. Dances were "the worst," according to this young woman, and she went to extremes to preserve her condition by paying another girl, who frequently dated her boy-friend's best friend, to show her where the women's room was and to tell her who was sitting where and dancing with whom.

There is a sort of spectrum of visibility. Thus, when this young woman received her first pair of contact lenses, she was able to jettison many of her protective antics, but still arose early every morning to put in her lenses before anyone else could see her. Later still, wearing long-term lenses, she could wear them to bed and wake up seeing. Her efforts at "face saving" are now limited to cleaning and sterilizing her lenses at a time when her boyfriend is certain to be elsewhere.

Bulimia, the "binge and purge" eating disorder, often leads its victims to organize their entire daily routine around the actions needed to carry out the "purging" aspect of their disorder in secrecy. One teen confided that she had broken off a very important relationship because the young man came to get her a half an hour early, thus forcing a postponement of her post-dinner vomiting.

LEVELS OF INTERACTION

We must also examine the levels of interaction in which the child participates, for the child may have different types of experiences at different levels. The film "Mask" showed the profound contrast between the child and his loving parent and their community of close friends and the cruelty of kids at the new high school and the parents of his summer camp friend. Often the home environment or the child's own imagination may be a warm haven to which he/she may retreat if stigmatizing incidents take place at other levels. Such is not always the case especially when parents are rejecting. John Merrick's mother sold him to the circus where he was kept in a cage, with no private place to go. Judging from what he told friends later in life, this remarkable man, by all accounts a gentle, kind and unembittered person, saved his sanity entirely by retreating into a world of memory and imagination, created by his considerable intelligence. In this way, he closed out the screams, jeers, and cruel remarks from the crowds who came to see him.

FAMILY-INFLICTED STIGMA

Although I have seen few cases, there are increasing numbers of children in our society whose appearance impairment is the result of abuse by a family member. Physical violence to the child with the intent to harm the child, not accidents or other situations in which a parent inadvertently causes injury to the child, fall under this rubric.

Obviously, a child who is deliberately victimized and whose appearance has been marred under those circumstances will suffer more psychological harm and will probably need psychotherapy for some time.

When I first met A., I thought he was one of the most beautiful children I had ever seen. He was just four years old, sturdily built, very black and had big intelligent eyes. He was super smart—a few of the staff had taught him to read when he was three—and he was demonstrative. He would come tearing down the hall, riding a free I.V. pole clutching a book. Then he would crawl into one's lap and begin to read. Sweet and jolly, but not always. Nightmares and fears plagued him.

For A.'s father had melted his hands in boiling water when A. was an infant because he "cried too much." He has had many operations to disengage his fingers. It was sad to hear people ask him what happened and to hear the response of his soft little voice: "My daddy melted my hands."

Recently, I visited the hospital where I first met A. almost twelve years ago. When I visited some old friends on the staff, I asked about him. He is still having operations and still in psychotherapy.

Obviously, to give adequate attention to children who have experienced almost unspeakable violence at the hands of people who should have been caring for them and raising them would require an entire book. We can merely note it as an important question for those interested in appearance impairment and for future research efforts. For the purposes of this book, it can be generally stated that here we have a child who scores strongly on almost every category of the model—strong support from loving foster parents and doting nurses, intelligence, a lovable personality, beautiful physical appearance (except the hands), humor, a consuming interest in reading and learning—but the trauma of the original event prevails over all these coping resources.

The Assessment Procedure

The assessment of a child can be accomplished by evaluation in terms of the major variables of the system, as depicted in Table 1 in the previous section. We examine each factor in terms of whether it helps or hinders the child in the struggle to avoid or cope with stigmatization and mark the result with a + or − beside the factor. We can thus see what areas of life are sources of strength for the child; in what areas the child may need help; and how well this child is doing compared to other children, especially those similar to him in other respects, such as age, gender, race, socio-economic class, and degree of physical damage to appearance. If the child can be assessed at different times during the treatment process, it can help us judge the effectiveness of therapy.

The categories in Table 1 can be described briefly as follows.

First, we must take as a given that all the children in this book, as Americans, experience the negative consequences of U.S. *culture* as set forth in Chapter Three. At the same time, we must also be alert to sub-cultural factors or the influence of other *ethnic cultures* that may have more positive views on impairment or be more humane in treating children. For example, in assessing Robert, in the following section (Table 5), we give him a − for U.S. culture, but add a + for Italian-American culture, because the latter emphasizes physical prowess and coordination in males of his age group—not just appearance.

The rest of the categories are those noted in our discussion of the model and shown in Figure 1 in Chapter Two.

Visibility is measured as "face" and "not face." Interviews with adults and children made it clear that facial stigma is by far the most worrisome to patients. Another reason for using this rather simple form of classification is the significance of the face in determining the nature of interpersonal interactions.

Levels of interaction refer to the different groups in which the child moves. First are close-knit, face-to-face groups like family, friendship groups, or gangs. Second are groups in which members have face-to-face knowledge of a person—they know who he or she is—but do not necessarily have a close relationship to the person. The class at school, members of one's church congregation, people in the neighborhood fall into this category. Finally, there are persons who are total strangers, such as someone seen on a bus or people who happen to be in the same restaurant as the person. We assign a + to the levels in which the child has support and with whom he or she feels comfortable. It is quite possible, for example, for a child to have a strong family support, while suffering teasing and cruelty in a new school.

Visually, the model for each child can be treated quantitatively with a + for each positive factor and a − for each negative factor. We can then add the pluses for an overall measure for each child. By organizing our assessment by general factors (e.g., "social resources") comprised of a number of more detailed factors (parental support, good survivor) and determining subtotals, we can identify areas of strength and of distress, and concentrate therapeutic measures where they are most needed. This approach also allows us to assess the child's feelings over time by comparing assessments carried out at different times.

APPLYING THE MODEL

The manner in which each child copes depends on the unique configuration, in his or her life, of all the factors noted in the model. In the ideal type of a positive coping situation of the child we would find:

A. A beneficial overall socio-cultural environment. Beauty would be less important in the society. Instead, kindness, courage, interactional ability would be revered. The religion would stress tolerance of the differences between people. Marriage would be based on character.

B. Visibility of the disfigurement would be minimal as would severity. Chances for repair would be good.

C. The child would be young (0–8) or in the late teens.

D. The child would have loving and supportive parents, and strong ties to extended kinship groups, religious congregation, neighborhood, and ethnic culture. He or she would have a few close and supportive friends. The parents would be upper or upper middle class, with educated and "important" connections.

E. The child would be intelligent, personable, and have a strong ego, good sense of humor, and an avid interest in some kind of talent or ability.

F. There would be a supportive ambiance. When a stigmatizing event occurs at level 3 or 4, there is ample reassurance at level 1 or 2.

In a "worst scenario":

A. Beauty would be of the greatest importance in the environment, and the appearance-impaired are not able to marry or attend school. The religion would view impairment as a sign of evil or of parental misdeeds.

B. The disfigurement would be highly visible, severe, and not repairable.

C. The child would be in the age range 9–13.

D. The child would be from a poor, lower caste, or lower class family with poor ties to community and kin. The parents would view the child as an embarrassment and not get along with one another very well. They might move frequently, subjecting the impaired child to too much change and transition.

E. The child would be of average or lower intelligence, not outgoing, with little sense of humor and pronounced talents, and would take little joy in any activity.

F. At each of the four levels of interaction, there would be little support for the child. People would make remarks on the street: in the ethnic community, people would pour out pity to the parents over the child's "condition"; and in school, no one in authority would stop teasing and taunting.

In this situation, there is no comfort, even within the family, because the parents view the child as the reason for their disgrace in the community.

Obviously these are the two most extreme situations. Most cases fall in between. Let us take a look at two typical cases from our study of skin disorders and apply this form of analysis to them.

Case of C.C.

C.C., a ten-year-old white female, has visible vitiligo on her face. It is *barely* visible, but it is there. The first signs appeared two summers ago when she was at camp. Her mother was quite shocked, upon visiting her over-night camp, to find the disorder all over the child's body.

The child was taken first to a doctor who said there was "no hope" in the treatment of vitiligo. Later they learned of a clinic. She has been going there (an Ivy League medical center with a vitiligo clinic) for over a year, but has not yet begun treatment, although the parents want her to begin. The child fears the treatment and broke into tears while talking with the doctor and nurse practitioner. She is afraid of the PUVA light and doesn't want to wear the sunglasses.

The vitiligo is not so bad during the winter because C.C. is very fair complexioned. However, during the summer, people at "the club" have asked questions and teased her. She also expressed fear about going back to camp this summer—especially about showering with other girls. At first, she was embarrassed "all the time" but says she doesn't let it bother her anymore. This is doubtless a "denial" statement as she broke down in tears while at the clinic and told of being taunted at school. So did her mother. The father seemed in control, but very *sad* about the daughter's situation. It is obvious that counseling would be a good idea. The child attends an elite private girls' school and there, too, she has experienced some incidents about vitiligo.

The upper class parents believe the child has become more, not less, upset about vitiligo, although they resist the interviewer's suggestion that she may be entering a pre-adolescent stage of general concern with appearance. The child's later outburst with the medical staff did indicate such a concern. Mother seemed quite ego-involved with the girl. When hearing of the child's emotional outburst, she immediately broke down herself.

Here we have a child of ten, just entering the period of concern with appearance and saddled with visible and spreading vitiligo on the face and legs. We see tremendous contradictions—statements of denial of effect coupled with tears. Denial of concern with appearance coupled with concern at wearing the sunglasses and "funny clothes" involved in treatment. Flat verbal statements coupled with extreme non-verbal gestures that signal emotional disturbance and nervousness.

Camp deserves a footnote. The girl dreads going this year as it was the place where onset of vitiligo occurred. There is some possibility that camp represents an exile from or rejection by parents.

Case of T.

Medical records indicate that T., a [then] eleven-year-old, Caucasian female presented at the clinic five years ago with vitiligo. The vitiligo started on the right lower quadrant, extending to both groins, extending to involve the legs. The vitiligo also appeared bilaterally on the arms. There is no family history of vitiligo or early graying according to the medical chart, but T. told the interviewer that several people on her mother's side have had prematurely gray hair. We interviewed the mother who appears to have black hair. In the daughter's interview, she stated that the mother also is prematurely gray. (One supposes that the mother dyes her hair.) There is no family history of nervous or endocrinological disorders. When seen again there had been some repigmentation on the knees and over the arms. A treatment of trisoralen was recommended. . . . The patient noted a return of pigment to many of the lesions on her shins and knees, even though she had missed quite a bit of her treatment during a camp session.

T. is extremely bright, articulate, and frank. She possesses a rich vocabulary, more like that of a college senior than a tenth grader. She wants to be an actress in the future and there is, along with this aim, a tendency to express ideas and emotions quite dramatically—not in the sense of being overly emotional—rather she simply does not leave one in doubt about her opinions and sentiments. She was not at all inhibited by the interview and is outspoken as well as open.

With considerable humor, T. described the onset of vitiligo. In this regard, she recalls that she thought this part of a normal developmental process. "I thought 'Well, when you're six, you get spots.'" It was her mother who became concerned upon visiting her at summer camp and noticing the spots. The mother was working at an "Ivy League" university a few years later, and not knowing that Dr. L. was a prominent authority in the field asked him to refer her to a dermatologist. He stated that he would see her himself.

This led to the first visit. Her treatment still consists of application of soralen and exposure to natural sun. There is now no visibility to her vitiligo.

In the interview she reports some embarrassing incidents of people staring at her or making unfortunate remarks. Her responses to this are direct—she tells people off. She tells them to shut up and she "told off" a counselor at her camp who went "Ew!" upon seeing her vitiligo. I asked her to assess her *feelings* about these events. Her response was (1) people who do make such remarks are "immature" and (2) "if people are going to judge me by my spots, they aren't worth having for friends. It's the same as prejudice."

She further observes that she has changed in her response. She says she "let it run my life for awhile," but now she doesn't let it get to her. She has supportive friends and family and she appreciates the relatively minor nature of her own case.

Observing her self and her self-image she says, "I may seem a paradigm of confidence, but I worry about many things." Immediately she linked this to her *age* rather than to the vitiligo. "People my age worry about appearance. They *all* think they have something wrong with them. They think they have acne, or they think their nose is too big or their eyes are too droopy. Vitiligo just falls into that category."

T's mother is an elegantly-attired New York architect who appears to be in her late 30s or early 40s. It is she who tells me about the onset of T.'s vitiligo and her own contact with Dr. L.

She believes T. is much more concerned about vitiligo as an adolescent than she was as a little girl. This is also what T. says, although T. sees herself as being on the upswing at this point. While the mother is concerned about T.'s worry about the disorder, she does believe it has caused T. to be more "religious" about her treatment.

The mother speaks out against medical persons who trivialize the disorder. She says that, from the start, her concern has been the possible psychological impact vitiligo might have on her daughter. She remembers with anger a pediatrician who told her to "forget it" as "nothing" could be done.

She discussed T.'s affection for Dr. L. and her full participation in all parts of the research which have resulted from it.

In summary, we have here an extremely bright, articulate, and attractive young woman who is able to share her responses to vitiligo with us through an introspective talent unusual in one of her age.

While she has had her worries and low points about vitiligo, it seems that a solid ego, zest for fun, intelligence, and a refusal to tolerate fools gladly all functioned in an adaptive fashion. There is no evidence of continued preoccupation with the disorder.

I believe her observations on the history of her responses to the disorder are extremely useful; we see the small child barely noticing the vitiligo, the young adolescent very concerned with it, the older adolescent emerging from this obsessive concern.

In assessing this patient's good coping, we must certainly keep in mind the relative invisibility of the vitiligo. The mother's anxiety plus the child's earlier concern indicate that, should the vitiligo spread, especially to the face, this effervescent aspiring actress could suffer psychological consequences.

SIMILARITIES AND DIFFERENCES BETWEEN T. AND C.C.

Despite the important differences to be discussed below, one is first struck by the similarities in the two cases. Both are young, white, and female. Both come from highly affluent families and can afford private schools and summer camps and skin clinics. In fact, the onset of both cases took place at summer camps, with startled mothers visiting their children and discovering the disfiguring disorder in the process. Both mothers report initial contacts with medical doctors as frustrating, with the physicians denying the significance of the disorder and/or seeming to be ignorant of modern treatments for the problem.

This set of common characteristics tells us a few things. Both girls have access to the finest, most recent therapeutic technology through family connections and wealth. Yet while T. has taken full advantage of the treatments, with some success in repair, C.C. has yet to begin treatment at all, expressing fear of the sunlamps and reluctance to don the requisite sunglasses.

It seems that T. has put the pessimism of the early doctors behind her, while C.C. took their statements to heart and sees herself as doomed to ugliness forever. Why?

One reason is age. C.C. is in the vulnerable pre-teen group, while T. is emerging from it. Another is the attitudes of the two mothers. While T.'s mother urges treatment and a focus on other aspects of life, C.C.'s mother is herself undone emotionally by her daughter's condition. While T.'s mother reminds her that many others are much less fortunate than she, C.C.'s mother weeps passive tears and doesn't even exert her influence to convince the girl to accept treatment. In addition, her attitude can surely reinforce the cultural stereotype of beauty as a female's only important trait.

In conversation with T., one becomes aware of the excitement and enthusiasm with which she imbues the future. She takes pride in her acting ability, her communication skills, and her intelligence. All of these are seen as valuable traits to be used in the development of her future life. In the case of C.C., no other assets were noted by the child or the parents and no talk took place about her future or her career— except for her mother's moaning, "But who will marry her?"

This suggests that we must be very careful to define what we mean by the term "family support," especially when we discuss it as a coping resource. On the surface, both girls seem to come from supportive family environments. The interviewer was impressed to see C.C.'s father at the clinic with his wife and child, as few fathers devote such time to their child's medical difficulties. Yet the concern of this family is one of intense—perhaps too intense—empathy and commiseration, rather than the supportive, "We know you can do it" concern of T.'s mother. Also, one cannot but note a more mature aspect to the concern of T.'s mother. In the interviewer's private discussion with her, we can see that she shares many of the cosmetically-oriented concerns expressed by C.C.'s parents. *But she does not wear these concerns on her sleeve and she does not bombard her child with them.* Rather, she has taken a matter-of-fact approach to treatment, and having done so, has set about a deliberate development of her daughter's self-esteem through encouragement and pride in her many other talents.

The effect of this strategy on T. has been positive, discouraging any attitude of self-sympathy or sense of hopelessness. We have here a child who is loved enough to have tremendous overall self-confidence, which we see not only in her happy approach to the future, but also in her present self-assurance and ability to "tell off" those who attempt to put her down. It is rare to see anger and "talking back" as responses to stigmatization attempts on children. We see denial, depression, and a myriad of other repressive responses. Yet, if people torment you, the really healthy response is to "tell them off," for it is their behavior which is at fault, not that of the victim. In fact, T. has always stood out in my memory, along with a few other tough kids, as one of the best copers I have known.

The tearful commiseration and apprehension of C.C.'s mother and the helpless worry-marks on her father's aristocratic face have not proven themselves as coping assets; instead they are liabilities. The message to the child is a negative one. Yes, she is loved—even doted upon—but she has the misfortune of being *pitied* within her family. The hidden message is "You are going to miss all the good things in life because you have a little (remember, the researcher described it as *barely* visible) discoloration on your face. Appearance is the most important factor in a woman's life. Your mother owes her happiness and good life to her beauty (remember, T.'s mother owes hers to being a successful professional) and mother weeps because she fears that your life will be miserable and sad because of what has happened to you."*

---

*This raises the summer camp factor again. It seems that the mothers may be responding differently to the events surrounding onset. While both may have experienced some guilt about this deforming event occurring in a context which has some aspects of parental abandonment, we saw no signs of this response in T.'s mother at this time, while the attitude of C.C.'s mother may well contain elements of continuing guilt. Certainly, many people, including child psychologists, believe that six is too young an age for overnight camp and its separation from parents, and there is a cultural notion that onset of vitiligo is often associated with emotional trauma. This association

Table 4 shows a comparative assessment of T. and C.C. This assessment confirms the interviewer's original impression of these cases. T. is very happy and well-adjusted. C.C. is in trouble.

T. has a high score (and C.C. a low one) in almost every area. The greatest difference lies in the area of *psychological resources*. This area is C.C.'s lowest point and might suggest the need for psychiatric help for C.C. and her family.

In order to see the value of our model in the effort to observe changes over time, let us re-examine the case of Robert, referred to earlier in this chapter. Table 5 compares his twelve-year-old profile to his present one. By the differences in the scores, we can see Robert's improvement. Furthermore, we can see that he has made good progress in psychological and social resources.

Another way of using the assessment measure might lie in the evaluation of treatment: assessing the child before treatment and again after it. Frances MacGregor, for instance, reports many positive changes following plastic surgery on children with cranial-facial disorders.[11]

Consider the case of Dawn, the myopic child discussed earlier. From an early age, she had to wear thick spectacles. She was ostracized by her classmates, who thought her retarded because of her appearance. No one invited her to a party or to join in sports activities. She scored very low on a modified version of the Coopersmith self-esteem measure.

Soft contact lenses in both eyes successfully corrected her vision. Table 6 compares her assessment at the time of the earlier interview with that based on an interview after she had worn the soft lenses for 6 weeks.

This analysis, admittedly crude, nonetheless shows a difference in the same child between two points in time, during which time she was presented with the technology needed to obliterate her stigma of

---

could lead to the mother's view that the vitiligo had been caused by her "rejection" of the child in sending to camp.

TABLE 4
Assessment: T. and C.C.

	T.	C.C.
U. S. Culture	−	−
Age	+	− (pre-teen)
Competency	+	−
Physiological Resources		
Visibility	+	− (on face)
Severity	−	−
Repairability	+	− (hasn't tried)
Psychological Resources		
Humor	+	−
Creativity	+	−
Intelligence	+	+
Friendliness	+	−
Self-esteem	+	−
Social Resources		
Parental support	+	+
Parental attitude	+	−
Parents' education	+	+
Wealth	+	+
Prestige/honor	+	+
Community/school involvement	+	−
Family stability	+	+
(Total)	(7)	(5)
Levels of Interaction		
Core—family, friends	+	−
Neighbors, acquaintances	+	−
Larger community	−	−
Unknown	−	−
(Total)	(2)	(0)
Total	18	6

TABLE 5
Assessment: Robert

	AGE 12	AGE 16
U. S. Culture	+[a]	+[a]
Age	−	+
Competency	−	+
Physiological Resources		
Visibility	−	−
Severity	−	−
Repairability	−	−
Psychological Resources		
Humor	−	+
Creativity	−	+
Intelligence	+	+
Friendliness	−	+
Self-esteem	−	+
Social Resources		
Parental support	+	+
Parental attitude	+	+
Parents' education	+	+
Wealth	−	−
Prestige/honor	−	−
Community/school involvement	+	+
Family stability	+	+
(Total)	(5)	(5)
Levels of Interaction		
Core—family, friends	+	+
Neighbors, acquaintances	+	+
Larger community	−	+
Unknown	−	−
(Total)	(2)	(3)
Total	9	16

[a]Italian-American

TABLE 6
Assessment: Dawn

	BEFORE CONTACT LENSES	AFTER CONTACT LENSES
U. S. Culture	−	−
Age	−	−
Competency	−	+
Physiological Resources		
Visibility	−	+
Severity	−	+
Repairability	−	+
Psychological Resources		
Humor	−	+
Creativity	−	+
Intelligence	+	+
Friendliness	−	+
Self-esteem	−	+
Social Resources		
Parental support	+	+
Parental attitude	+	+
Parents' education	+	+
Wealth	−	−
Prestige/honor	−	−
Community/school involvement	+	+
Family stability	+	+
(Total)	(5)	(5)
Levels of Interaction		
Core—family, friends	+	+
Neighbors, acquaintances	−	+
Larger community	−	+
Unknown	−	+
(Total)	(1)	(4)
Total	7	18

heavy "Coke-bottle-bottom" spectacles. We can see first the overall gain; then note that she has improved the most in the areas of "psychological" and "levels of interaction" resources. She has acquired humor, self-esteem, and competency through the interaction of her new, pretty "self" with family and friends; their approval has made her more outgoing.

We also note many changes from negative to positive in the section on physiological factors: the contact lenses have eliminated visibility and severity of disfigurement, essentially eliminating the cause of past stigmatization. In essence, this is no longer a child with impaired appearance and all the other changes arise from that fact.

Few are as fortunate as Dawn in the availability of an "overnight" elimination of stigma; some must patiently endure months or years of treatment and there are still many for whom no treatment or cure exists. Those children must set upon the painful path of acceptance, of facing life as a freak and trying to salvage from it what dignity, acceptance, and joy they can.

There is more we can do for all children who suffer an impaired appearance. As well as efforts to eliminate the impairments, we can work on other facets of the problem—the flagging ego of the child, the education of the general population on the *facts* associated with impairment, efforts to deal with media and other cultural purveyors of stereotypes about impaired appearance, and a recommitment to a kinder, more-caring set of values.

Coping Strategies

So far, we have used an ordinal approach to children's efforts to handle the situation of impaired appearance. Like Pearlin, we see these efforts as "better than" or "worse than" others and we have indicated that the more positive resources a child has available, the better he or she is able to cope with impaired appearance.

Now we will examine the tactics children may employ in the

coping process from a *nominal* perspective. That is, while these tactics differ from one another, there is no ranking or comparative measurement among them. A denier is no "better" or "worse" than an intellectualizer: simply different. The coping measures one sees children with impaired appearance employ tend to fall into these categories: denial, intellectualization, anger, depression/withdrawal, education.

INTELLECTUALIZATION

In intellectualization, the child copes by (1) identifying with the physicians rather than with fellow patients, and (2) intellectualizing the causes and prognosis of the impairment. Thus some emotional distance is created between the child and the impairment. The child backs away from the disorder, as if he or she were a medical person studying it, not a victim suffering from it.

Steve was born with very short arms and unformed hands. In a series of operations, doctors hoped to at least create a thumb oppositional to the other, fused fingers. His parents had travelled abroad during the time that the mother was pregnant with Steve and she had taken thalidomide while in Europe. It was believed that this was the cause of the impairment. He was eleven when we met, awaiting further surgery. He told many stories of being teased or ridiculed, especially on the street. He attended Catholic school, and he told me that the nuns would not tolerate taunting of this nature.

Very bright, Steve had become an authority on his condition. He read about it in popular and medical journals. His many trips to the hospital had resulted in his familiarity with medical jargon and procedure. Often he surprised doctors with the extent of his knowledge.

ANGER

Anger is perhaps the most honest form of coping strategy in that it acknowledges the fact of stigma, protests the unfairness of stigma distribution (Why me?) and strikes back at those who attempt to derogate one by stigmatization.

Yet it is not a common coping strategy. This fact is not so strange as we initially might suppose. Children in our society are often trained to be "seen but not heard." They are also told to "turn the other cheek" or to "be a sport" when people say rude things or ridicule them. In addition, they are taught never to talk back to adults. Thus, when adults make remarks or point their fingers, most children remain silent, repressing their anger in respect for the social norms of politeness.

But not all children hold back. We saw above, in the case of T., that if people "hassle" her, she "tells them off." We also see some of the male children respond with rage and/or profanity. This is quite rare among girls, however, who are being socialized for adulthood, which in our culture means never to show anger, always to think of the other person's feelings, and to repress all negative feelings.

DEPRESSION/WITHDRAWAL

One result of repressed anger is depression. The taboo against showing anger or directing one's anger against another leads to repression of that anger which is ultimately directed inward against the self.

C.C. earlier in this chapter exemplifies this tendency. Although she has many coping resources—wealth, concerned parents, intelligence, community status—she is depressed. She has been brought up to be exceptionally polite under all circumstances and there is no acceptable vehicle for the articulation of anger. She accepts society's judgment of her appearance.

Withdrawal is seen quite often among adults with impaired appearance, but less often in children, as it is a form of behavior often forbidden the child. As we have previously noted, children cannot refuse to attend school, although adults can choose to become recluses. The laws governing public education alone make this coping strategy non-optional for children.

EDUCATION

We noted above the tendency of mothers of children with impaired appearance to attempt to educate their tormentors. In the story of mother and daughter having their pre-Christmas spree ruined by peering strangers, we saw the mother use education as a means of coping with her child's humiliation.

The benefits of this approach are many: by taking the educative role, one places oneself above the inflicters of stigma (the educator is above conflict and name calling). Also, there is a chance that the message will really reach the other parties and thus convert them. It also wins the approval of doctors.

Several of the children with whom I have worked used this strategy:

> A five-year-old black girl with vitiligo all around her mouth tells us, "My mother said, just tell them it is pigment cells dying. It isn't catching and it doesn't hurt."

Chapter 6

Epilogue: Doing Something

> The psychic scars caused by believing that you are ugly
> leave a permanent mark on your personality.
>
> Joan Rivers, quoted by Lydia Lane

Recent Gains

The establishment of a variety of foundations that take up the cause of the appearance-impaired is encouraging. The Sturges-Weber Foundation, Let's Face It, the International Foundation for Craniofacial Disorders, and the Frontiers Vitiligo Association are examples. The groups supply general educational material on particular disorders, advise patients and their families, carry out research, and provide emotional support. Some organizations, such as Let's Face It of New England, have been established by and for the victims themselves.

The success of "Phantom of the Opera" on Broadway and "Beauty and the Beast" on television may be indicative of a more open attitude of the public toward people with impaired appearance.

An interesting innovation has been the introduction of fictional characters with appearance impairments and physical handicaps into the children's general cultural milieu. Several of the new characters on "Sesame Street" have what we would call stigmatizing conditions, and a new group of puppets all of whom are appearance-impaired are making appearances all over the country.

Most surprising and quite amazing is a commercial for one of

America's most famous fast food restaurants. It depicts the animated interaction between two teenaged girls on their way to lunch, and concludes with the girls sitting down with two young men at the restaurant. It is only halfway through the commercial, as the girls approach the restaurant, that we realize that one of them is in a wheelchair.

What can we do to make the lives of children with impaired appearance better? Our observations of the effectiveness and ineffectiveness of coping strategies and a consideration of the factors that better or worsen the child's situation of impairment suggest some courses of action to us.

Better Assessment of Children's Situations

People must carefully examine each child's case in terms of his or her ability to cope with stigmatization and objectification.

The cases to which we applied our assessment model at the end of the last chapter suggest the utility of applying *qualitative* as well as *quantitative* measures in our efforts to assist children with impaired appearance. One could have been content with "scoring" T's and C.C.'s reactions, by assigning a score of + 1 for every coping asset and a score of − 1 for every coping deficit and then giving each girl a Composite Coping Index Score, but I believe it would have afforded us and the patients little. For one thing, their many similarities (age, class, gender, etc.) mean that the two scores might have been quite similar. Given the problems of motherly overinvolvement and some facial vitiligo, C.C. would probably receive a "lower" coping score. But so what? It would not tell us much about what her difficulties are or how to help her.

A qualitative measure allows us to develop an idea of *where* the strengths and weaknesses lie in the child's coping repertoire. We can then reinforce the strengths and get to work *appropriately* on the weaknesses.

An analysis of the case of Rory, a youth of sixteen with pronounced facial vitiligo, illustrates this point.

This black youth has vitiligo of an extreme nature on his head, face, hands, mustache and neck. This is one of the most marked cases the researcher has seen, and it is completely unilateral. That is, the right side of his face is an attractive solid brown-black color; and then, as if a line has been drawn right down his face, the left side is pied—with patches of vitiligo. This condition started after a kidney infection. He is a new patient at H. clinic and just starting treatment, so no report can be made on the progress of repigmentation.

He seems a classic denier. Throughout the interview he disclaimed any concern about the condition, repeatedly saying, "I don't let it bother me." In view of the fact that he has undergone a complete transformation from a handsome young man into a deformed one in less than two months, this statement seems highly doubtful.

He acknowledges that some people stare at him, but says, "I just keep on doing what I'm doing." He says nothing has changed at school. "Everybody sees me as the same old person, they are my buddies." He says his mother is also a good friend with whom he can discuss "anything."

He thinks teachers should realize that vitiligo patients may be "scared and nervous." He says, "Teachers should talk to other kids about vitiligo so they don't hurt the victims."

He refuses to consider cosmetics, as, "A man don't wear makeup."

This is one of the saddest cases seen during the study. The contrast between his movie-star handsome right side and his bizarre left side is sobering. Treatment may, in fact, repigment this young man in time, but during the interim, some effort must be made to reach him at the psychological level. His denial is strong, his emotions flat. The only real key is when we asked him what he would advise teachers, he replied, "The vitiligo patient may be scared and nervous."

Considered quantitatively, the use of denial here might be misleading, for he answers most of the interviewer's question "correctly," that is, the way he thinks they ought to be answered. He claims to have no problems with stigmatization, appears to be doing well, but the remark about the victim as "scared and nervous" tips us off, as does his statement that males do not wear make-up.

A qualitative approach suggests a session with a male cosmetologist to show how well his condition can be hidden, and perhaps a conversation between doctor and mother on fear. The male friendship network sounds like a good source of support and should be encouraged.

Similarly C.C.'s case need not be assessed as "better" or "worse" than T.'s. Use of our assessment technique would simply pinpoint the weak areas, and help us address them.

A Word to Professionals

It is very important that all professionals understand the far-reaching social and psychological consequences of impaired appearance on the life of the child. Too often one sees this aspect of the situation trivialized or ignored. Physicians, nurses, social workers must all gain a better understanding of how critically important appearance is to children and their peers. How easy it is for us, as adults, to forget this aspect of our youth, especially the early adolescent years!

Nor is it only medical people who need to acquire greater sensitivity in this area. Over and over again, I have been shocked by stories of school teachers who ignore the cruelty of children to their impaired classmates, who condone it, and who take part in it themselves. Most recently, a child who had an eye removed told of being harassed, teased, and hit on the school bus while neither the driver nor a teacher riding the bus intervened. It must be made perfectly clear that not acting in such a situation constitutes approval.

We have seen that many appearance-impaired children feel that their situation has been trivialized. When they have voiced concerns to their doctors, they have often been told that they should "stop feeling sorry for themselves." Doctors, nurses, teachers, and social workers must realize that these children suffer from embarrassment, shame, and depression as a result of their appearance.

An understanding adult professional can deal with mild psychological reactions by being a good listener and giving some advice on treatment and the use of cosmetics to camouflage the disorder.

Cosmetics *are* useful to many patients as a concealment strategy. Some individuals find special dermatological cosmetics effective; others are satisfied with a mixture of over-the-counter brands. If patients are concerned about their appearance, they should be encouraged to experiment with a wide range of cosmetics.

These children worry about the social impact of their disorder. They are concerned about the unknown side effects of treatment. They worry about the genetic aspects of the disease: will they pass it on to children and grandchildren? These worries tend to build and intensify if they are repressed. A recent study found that although the majority of the vitiligo patients surveyed had questions and anxieties about their condition, only a minority had voiced these concerns to their doctors. People said that their doctors were always in a hurry, abrupt, or seemingly uninterested in the patient. We must encourage appearance-impaired children to ask questions and to discuss their concerns. To do this, we must respond positively to the questions they do ask, or they will repress deeper concerns.

One should carefully evaluate the individual children's emotional reaction to impairment giving them additional support or reassurance. For more severe emotional reactions, referral to psychiatric personnel for individual or group therapy is helpful.

The child patient with impaired appearance needs special attention, especially the junior-high-school-age child. During the preteen and early teen years, appearance assumes great importance. Young children may be protected from some of the negative psychological consequences by supportive parents and by developing competencies in other areas, but even for the elementary-school child, periods of transition (such as moving or going to a new school) may be particularly stressful. Children should be evaluated for stress. Reassurance or encouragement to develop competency in other areas is helpful to many children. Children who seem disturbed by the disorder may need individual or group psychiatric therapy.

It is important to evaluate the child without the presence of the parent. Parents may sometimes try to protect the child by denying the child's psychic distress, or in some cases, children may avoid describing their true feelings to protect the parent.

American society places a high value on appearance. Numerous studies have documented the preference for attractive people in school grading, friend selection, and help in emergency situations. The child who fears the social consequences of impaired appearance is not paranoid, but responding to a very real situation in our society. This fact should underlie our dealings with children whose appearance has been impaired.

Public Education

The work done by many recent researchers, especially on maternal behavior toward infants born with impaired appearance, suggests a vital need for public education about the origins, future prognosis, and treatment of congenital appearance disorders and about the universal need of each child, *regardless of appearance,* for unqualified parental love, touch, and support.

In fact, loving support during the first days of life may be the most vital contribution parents can make: work with older children and adults supports the idea that those who acquire a strong ego and sense of personhood during early life are much better able to cope with impaired appearance as older children and adults.

Values Reevaluated

Concerned people must launch and continue a culture-wide attack on our society's over-concern with and adulation of superficial beauty, at the cost of concern with deeper traits. In raising our children, we must put appearance low on the list, stressing character, intelligence, kindness, and creativity over "prettiness," for in twentieth-century America *normal* children are objectified, categorized, and dehumanized because of their age status. In Chapter Three we examined some of the ways in which children are slighted, exploited, and abused *as children*. When we add to this the burden of impaired appearance, we create a situation of double stigma. The child bears *two* negative statuses: that of a child and that of a person with impaired appearance. Until we begin to deal with children as real people, as long as we view and treat our children as projections of ourselves and our dreams, or as possessions which help us display our accomplishments, we are treating them as objects, and those bearing the signs of "imperfection" are treated as damaged objects.

Those who work intimately with appearance impaired children, like MacGregor, the Salyers, and Betsy Wilson at Let's Face It, know how deeply the condition of stigma can affect a child and how far into adulthood that influence extends. Yet I know from conversations with my academic and medical colleagues that many of them think I am exaggerating or reacting oversensitively to the children's plight.

How can I convince such skeptics? Actually, one of my university colleagues inadvertently showed me a way. We were discussing our research projects over coffee one afternoon, when my colleague, a very pretty woman, shook her head and told me that "No one's whole personality could be influenced just by looking funny. I'm sure most people just adapt to that kind of thing in time, and don't think much about it." I rather vehemently disagreed, and our conversation shifted to the mysteries of the new computer which was being installed in the business school.

A week later, I received a phone call from my colleague, canceling our weekly lunch by the "Bio frog pond." She had an apology to make. A few days after our conversation, a bee had stung her on the upper lip. Her lip had swollen to twice its normal size and was also discolored. She described it as "one of the worst things" that has ever happened to her. People stared at her on the first day, some asked her if her husband had hit her. Others just gaped. A typical scholar, she owned no make-up, but had purchased some in an effort to hide or minimize the bite. While the foundation covered the purple color, it could not diminish the swelling; she still looked disfigured. Finally, "I decided I just can't go anywhere until this goes away. You were right. It's mortifying, I've asked Y. (husband and fellow professor) to take my classes and I've bowed out of all our social obligations until it goes down."

There is a saying, part of Native American wisdom though reduced to a cliché by whites who like to write it on pieces of bark and sell for souvenirs, in which there remains an element of uncheapened, untacky truth: Let me not judge another until I have walked a mile in his moccasins. Walking in the moccasins of the appearance-impaired had literally turned this woman around and sensitized her to the problems, pains, and anxieties experienced by stigmatized people. And it suggested a learning tactic to me.

Here is a simple task that anyone can do. Locate a theatrical supply company or costumer in your town or city. There you will find, in glass cases, an abundant supply of fake birthmarks, growths, scars, bleeding lesions, warts, and welts. Buy one. When you get home, put it on your face and then go somewhere you have recently or routinely been (for example, ride the same bus or train you usually take to work, ask a friend to lunch at a restaurant where you are a "regular," pick up your child at the school bus stop). Keep a written or taped record of the events that transpire and your reaction to these. I'm sure you will find it a truly educative experience.

I began this book with the story of a ten-year-old child, who, tormented by his classmates about his chubbiness, committed suicide in his elementary school classroom. It should never have happened. But it did. Societal attitudes and values, major institutions, and authority figures supported the classmate's contemptuous attitudes, the child was entering that point in the life-cycle when appearance is most highly valued. He had no high statuses to countervail his being a child and a not-beautiful person. His self-esteem had taken such a beating that he had few psychological coping resources available to him. He had access to firearms. In a way, it was bound to happen.

That boy and his action confirmed my desire to write this book. Let those of you who read it join me in a rededication of ourselves to the cause of the appearance-impaired child. Let us think, speak, and act toward the accomplishment of a single, simple goal: that this may never happen again.

Appendix: Caring Organizations

This list of organizations concerned with issues related to impaired appearance is current as of January 1990.

Craniofacial Center
Children's Hospital of Boston
300 Longwood Ave.
Boston, MA 02115
617-735-6309   Contact: Kathryn Morent

International Craniofacial Foundation
10210 North Central Expressway, LB 37
Dallas, TX 75231
800-535-3643   Contact: Dr. Marcy Rogers

Institute for Identity and Body Image
Box 98048
Houston, TX 77048
703-790-7702

Let's Face It
Box 711
Concord, MA 01742
508-371-3186   Contact: Betsy Wilson

National Neurofibromatosis Foundation, Inc.
141 Fifth Ave. Suite 7-S
New York, NY 10010
800-323-7938

National Stroke Association
1420 Ogden St.
Denver, CO 80218
303-839-1992

Sturges-Weber Foundation
P.O. Box 460931
Aurora, CO 80015
303-693-2986   Contact: Karen L. Ball

Vitiligo Group
P.O. Box 919
London SE21 8AW, England
01-670-7175   Contact: Sarojini Ariyanayagam

Notes

Chapter Two

1. Aaron Lerner and James Nordlund, "Vitiligo: What is it? Is it Important?" *JAMA* 239 (1978): 1183–89.

2. A. Adler, *Study of Organ Inferiority and Its Physical Compensations* (New York: Nervous and Mental Disease Publishing Company, 1917); Claire H. Liachowitz, *Disability as a Social Construct: Legislative Roots* (Philadelphia: University of Pennsylvania Press, 1988).

3. R. Barker, B. Wright, L. Meyerson, and M. Gonick, *Adjustment to Physical Handicaps and Illness: A Survey of the Social Psychology of Physical Disability* (New York: Social Science Research Council, 1953), Bulletin 53; Daryl Bem, *Beliefs, Attitudes, and Human Affairs* (Belmont, Ca.: Brooks/Cole, 1970); L. Centers and R. Centers, "Peer Group Attitudes Toward the Amputee Child," *Journal of Social Psychology* 61 (1963): 127–32; R. Johnson and L. Heal, "Private Employment Agency Responses to the Physically Handicapped," *Journal of Applied Rehabilitation Counseling* 7 (1976): 12–21; N. Goodman, S. Dornbusch, S. Robinson, and A. Hastorf, "Variant Reactions to Physical Disabilities," *American Sociological Review* 28 (1963): 429–35.

4. E. J. Langer *et al.*, "Stigma, Staring, and Discomfort: A Novelty Stimulus Hypothesis," *Journal of Experimental Psychology* 12 (1976): 451–63.

5. T. Cash, B. Gillen, and D. Burns, "Sexism and Beautyism in Personal Consultant Decision Making," *Journal of Applied Psychology* 62 (1977): 301–10.

6. J. Wolfgang and A. Wolfgang, "Personal Space: An Unobtrusive Measure of Attitudes Toward the Physically Handicapped," *Proceedings of the 76th Annual Convention of the American Psychological Association* 3 (1968): 653–54.

7. Johnson and Heal, *op. cit.*

8. V. Christopherson, "Role Modification of the Disabled Male," *American Journal of Nursing* 68 (1968): 290–93.

9. H. Doob and B. Ecker, "Stigma and Compliance," *Journal of Personality and Social Psychology* 14 (1970): 302–04; J. Dwyer and J. Meyer, "Psychological Effects of Variation in Physical Appearance During Adolescence," *Adolescent* 3 (1968–69): 353–58; S. Taylor and W. Reitz, *The Three Faces of*

Self-Esteem, Department of Psychology, University of Western Ontario Research Bulletin 80 (1968).

10. *New York Times,* November 16, 1980, p. 22E.

11. F. Whitlock, *Psychophysiological Aspects of Skin Disorder* (London: W. B. Saunders, 1976).

12. Gordon Allport, *The Nature of Prejudice* (Garden City, N.Y.: Doubleday-Anchor, 1958).

13. Howard S. Becker, *Outsiders: Studies in the Sociology of Deviance* (New York: Free Press, 1963); Thomas Scheff, *Being Mentally Ill* (Chicago: Aldine, 1966); David Matza, *Delinquency and Drift* (New York: John Wiley, 1964).

14. John Lofland, *Deviance and Identity* (Englewood Cliffs, N.J.: Prentice-Hall, 1969), p. 22.

15. Scheff, *op. cit.;* Edwin M. Schur, *Labeling Women Deviant: Gender, Stigma, and Social Control* (New York: Random House, 1984), pp. 30–34; Becker, *op. cit.;* Erving Goffman, *Stigma: Notes on the Management of Spoiled Identity* (Englewood Cliffs, N.J.: Prentice-Hall, 1963).

16. Becker, *op. cit.*

17. Schur, *op. cit.*

18. *Ibid.*

19. Edwin M. Lemert, *Social Pathology* (New York: McGraw-Hill, 1951), p. 77.

20. Karen Dion, "What is Beautiful is Good," *Journal of Personality and Social Psychology* 24 (1972): 215–20; and "Physical Attractiveness and the Evaluation of Children's Transgressions," *Journal of Personality and Social Psychology* 24 (1972): 207–13.

21. Dion, *op. cit.;* A. Miller, "The Role of Physical Attractiveness in Impression Formation," *Psychonomic Science* 19 (1970): 241–53; A. Miller, "Social Perception and Internal/External Control," *Perceptual and Motor Skills* 30 (1970): 103–09; Centers and Centers, *op. cit.;* Janice Mercer, Henry Andrews, and Arthur Mercer, "The Effects of Physical Attractiveness and Disability on Client Ratings by Helping Professionals," *Journal of Applied Rehabilitation Counseling* (1983): 41–45.

22. T. Cash, J. Kehr, J. Polyson, and V. Freeman, "The Role of Physical Attractiveness in Peer Attribution of Psychological Disturbance," *Journal of Consulting and Clinical Psychology* 45 (1977): 987–93; Allport, *op. cit.*

23. Goffman, *op. cit.,* p. 19.

24. Allport, *op. cit.*

25. S. McKelvie and J. Matthews, "Effects of Physical Attractiveness and Favorableness of Character on Liking," *Psychological Reports* 38 (1976): 1223–30.

26. E. Berscheid, E. Walster, and G. Bohrenstedt, "The Happy Body: A Survey Report," *Psychology Today* 6 (1973): 119–31; T. Cash and P. Begley, "Internal-External Control, Achievement Orientation, and Physical Attractiveness," *Psychology Reports* 38 (1976): 1205–06; Cash, Gillan, and Burns, *op. cit.;* Cash, Hehr, Polyson, and Freeman, *op. cit.;* Dion, *op. cit.;* D. Landy and H. Sigall, "Beauty is Talent: Task Evaluation as a Function of the Performer's Physical Attractiveness," *Journal of Personality and Social Psychology* 29 (1974): 299–304; Miller, *op. cit.;* R. Barocas and F. Vance, "Physical Appearance and Personal Adjustment to Counselling," *Journal of Consulting and Clinical Psychology* 21 (1974): 96–100.

27. David Grey and Richard Ashmore, "Blasing Influence on Sentencing: Characteristics of Simulated Sentencing," *Psychology Reports* 38, 1 (June 1976): 727–38.

28. J. Schwartz and S. Abramonitz, "Effects of Female Client Physical Attractiveness on Clinical Judgement," *Psychotherapy: Theory, Research, and Practice* 15 (1978): 251–57.

29. Sheila Dietz, Madeleine Littman, and Brenda Bentley, "Attribution of Responsibility for Rape: The Influences of Observer Empathy, Victim Resistance, and Victim Attractiveness," *Sociology of Sex Roles* 10 (Feb. 1984): 260–80.

30. Centers and Centers, *op. cit.;* J. Siller, L. Ferguson, D. Vann, and B. Holland, "The Structure of Attitudes Toward the Physically Disabled: The Disability Factor Scale: Amputation, Blindness, Cosmetic Conditions," *Proceedings of the 76th Annual Convention of the American Psychological Association* 3 (1978): 251–57; Robert Kleck, "Physical Stigma and Non-Verbal Cues Emitted in Face-to-Face Interaction," *Human Relations* 21 (1968): 19–28; S. Fugita, T. Agie, I. Newman, and N. Walfish, "Attractiveness, Self-Concept and a Methodological Note About Gaze," *Personality and Social Psychology Bulletin* 3 (1977): 240–43; Siller *et al., op. cit.;* C. J. VanderKolk, "Physiological Measures as a Means of Assessing Reactions to the Disabled," *New Outlook for the Blind* 70 (1976): 101–03.

31. Centers and Centers, *op. cit.;* Dion, *op. cit.* (1972a;b).

32. Barocas and Vance, *op. cit.;* Centers and Centers, *op. cit.;* Johnson and Heal, *op. cit.*

33. L. J. Pillavin *et al.,* "Costs, Diffusion, and the Stigmatized Victim," *Journal of Personality and Social Psychology* 32 (1975): 429–38.

34. Cynthia Kmiecik, Paula Mausar, and George Banzinger, "Attractiveness and Interpersonal Space," *Journal of Social Psychology* 108 (Aug. 1979): 277–78.

35. Allport, *op. cit.*

36. Fugita *et al.*, *op. cit.*

37. Schur, *op. cit.*

38. Becker, *op. cit.*

39. *Ibid.*, p. 33.

40. Schur, *op. cit.*, p. 24.

41. *Ibid.*; Scheff, *op. cit.*; David Sudnow, "Normal Crimes," *Social Problems* 12 (Winter 1965): 255–76; J. P. Wiseman, *The Lively Commerce* (New York: Signet Books, 1972).

42. Schur, *op. cit.*, pp. 30–34.

43. Allport, *op. cit.*, p. 14.

44. Schur, *op. cit.*

45. Earl Rubington and Martin S. Wineberg, eds., *Deviance: The Interactionist Perspective* (New York: Macmillan, 1987).

46. Scheff, *op. cit.*; Becker, *op. cit.*; Matza, *op. cit.*; Schur, *op. cit.*

47. Frances Cooke MacGregor, *Transformation and Identity: The Face and Plastic Surgery* (Oak Grove, Ill.: Eterna Press, 1980); S. Shuster, G. Fisher, E. Harris, and D. Binnell, "The Effects of Skin Diseases on Self-Image," *British Journal of Dermatology* 99 (1978): 18–19; J. Dixon, "Coping with Prejudice: Attitudes of Handicapped Persons Toward the Handicapped," *Journal of Chronic Disease* 30 (1977): 307–22; Landy, *op. cit.*; Barker, *et al.*, *op. cit.*; Whitlock, *op. cit.*

48. Allport, *op. cit.*

49. Beatrice A. Wright, *Physical Disability: A Psychosocial Approach* (New York: Harper and Row, 1960, second edition 1983).

50. J. Money and E. Pollet, "Studies in the Psychology of Dwarfism," *Journal of Pediatrics* 68 (1966): 391–96.

51. L. J. Pearlin and Carma Schooler, "The Structure of Coping," *Journal of Health and Social Behavior* 32 (1978): 2–21.

52. J. C. Ventimiglia, "Sex Roles and Chivalry: Some Conditions to Altruism," *Sociology of Sex Roles* 8 (Nov. 1982): 1107–22.

53. Steven Hobfoll and Louis Pennerm, "Effect of Physical Attractiveness on Therapists' Initial Judgments of a Person's Self-Concept," *Journal of Consulting and Clinical Psychology* 46 (Feb. 1978): 200–201.

54. Goffman, *op. cit.*, p. 38.

55. Schur, *op. cit.*, p. 38.

56. Dietz, *op. cit.*; F. Davis, "Deviance Disavowal: The Management of Strained Interaction by the Visibly Handicapped," *Social Problems* 9 (1961): 120–32; Grey and Ashmore, *op. cit.*

57. Scheff, *op. cit.*; Matza, *op. cit.*; Schur, *op. cit.*

58. Goffman, *op. cit.*, p. 7.

59. Pearlin and Schooler, *op. cit.*, p. 21.
60. *Ibid.*
61. *Ibid.*, p. 5.
62. *Ibid.*
63. *Ibid.*
64. *Ibid.*

Chapter Three

1. Hilda Bruch, *Eating Disorders: Anorexia Nervosa, Obesity, and the Person Within* (New York: Basic Books, 1973), p. 14.
2. *Ibid.* See also S. Cloete, "I Speak for the African," *Life* 34 (1973): 111.
3. Ralph Linton, *The Study of Man* (New York: Appleton-Century, 1936).
4. Elaine Showalter, *The Female Malady: Women, Madness and English Culture, 1830–1890* (New York: Penguin, 1984), p. 107.
5. Daryl Bem, *Beliefs, Attitudes, and Human Affairs* (Belmont, Ca.: Brooks/Cole, 1970).
6. Marcia Millman, *Such a Pretty Face: Being Fat in America* (New York: W. W. Norton, 1980).
7. Joseph E. Murray, John Mulliken, Leonard Kapan, and Myron Belfer, "Twenty Year Experience in Maxillo-Craniofacial Surgery," *Annals of Surgery* 190, 3 (Sept. 1979): 320–31.
8. Kenneth Salyer, Marcy Rogers-Salyer, and Members of the Texas Craniofacial Center, *Craniofacial Deformity: A Booklet for Parents*, 3rd ed. (Dallas: Texas Foundation for Craniofacial Deformities, 1985).
9. *Ibid.*
10. Gerhard Lenski and Jean Lenski, *Human Societies*, 6th ed. (New York: McGraw-Hill, 1982), pp. 161, 208, 341, 378–79. See also Vivian A. Zelizer, *Pricing the Priceless Child: The Changing Social Value of Children* (New York: Basic Books, 1985).
11. Philippe Ariès, *Centuries of Childhood: A Social History of Family Life*, trans. by Robert Baldick (New York: Vintage Books, 1962).
12. Zelizer, *op. cit.*
13. Jeffrey G. Fleishman and Carol Cleveland, "Broken Children," Allentown, Pa. *Morning Call*, Nov. 1987, #35, 116, p. 4.
14. Ann Hill Beuf, *Biting Off the Bracelet: A Study of Children in Hospitals*, 2nd ed. (Philadelphia: University of Pennsylvania Press, 1989). See also Zelizer, *op. cit.*
15. Frances Cooke MacGregor, *Transformation and Identity: The Face and*

Plastic Surgery (Oak Grove, Ill.: Eterna Press, 1980). MacGregor's work became known to me only after the major part of this book was completed. Nonetheless, I found it of great help, and appreciate the consistency of my observations with hers.

Chapter Four

1. Frances Cooke MacGregor, *Transformation and Identity: The Face and Plastic Surgery* (Oak Grove, Ill.: Eterna Press, 1980).

2. Kenneth Salyer, Marcy Rogers-Salyer, and Members of the Texas Craniofacial Center, *Craniofacial Deformity: A Booklet for Parents,* 3rd ed. (Dallas: Texas Foundation for Craniofacial Deformities, 1985).

3. Leslie A. Fiedler, *Freaks: Myths and Images of the Secret Self* (New York: Simon and Schuster, 1978).

4. "The Quiet Revolution" (Association for the Care of Children in Hospitals).

5. Material supplied by Texas Craniofacial Center, Dallas.

6. Marcy Rogers-Salyer, A. Gayle Jensen, and Christopher Borden, "Effects of Facial Deformities and Physical Attractiveness on Mother-Infant Bonding," in *Craniofacial Surgery: Proceedings of the First International Congress of the International Society of Cranio-Maxillo-Facial Surgery* (1985).

7. *Ibid.*

8. K. Salyer, *et al., op. cit.*

9. Erik Erikson, *Childhood and Society,* 2nd ed. rev. (New York: W. W. Norton, 1968).

10. Erving Goffman, *Stigma: Notes on the Management of Spoiled Identity* (Englewood Cliffs, N.J.: Prentice-Hall, 1963).

Chapter Five

1. L. J. Pearlin and Carma Schooler, "The Structure of Coping," *Journal of Health and Social Behavior* 32 (1978): 2–21.

2. Erving Goffman, *Stigma: Notes on the Management of Spoiled Identity* (Englewood Cliffs, N.J.: Prentice-Hall, 1963).

3. Frances Cooke MacGregor, *Facial Deformities and Plastic Surgery* (New York: Charles Thomas, 1953).

4. Erik Erikson, *Childhood and Society,* 2nd ed. rev. (New York: W. W. Norton, 1968).

5. E. Berscheid, E. Walster, and G. Bohrenstedt, "The Happy Body: A Survey Report," *Psychology Today* 6 (1973): 119–31.

6. J. Dwyer and J. Meyer, "Psychological Effects of Variation in Physical Appearance During Adolescence," *Adolescent* 3 (1968–69): 353–58.

7. Berscheid *et al., op. cit.*

8. Arlene Skolnick, "The Myth of the 'Vulnerable Child,'" *Psychology Today* (Feb. 1978): 55–60, 65.

9. Erikson, *op. cit.*

10. Judith Porter, Ann Hill Beuf, James Nordlund, and Aaron Lerner, "Personal Responses of Patients to Vitiligo," *Archives of Dermatology* 114 (1978): 1384–85; Ann Hill Beuf and Judith Porter, "Children Coping with Impaired Appearance: Social and Psychological Influences," *General Hospital Psychiatry* 6 (Oct. 1984): 294–301.

11. MacGregor, *op. cit.*

Bibliography

Abram, R. "Psychology of Chronic Illness." *Journal of Chronic Diseases* 25 (1972): 659–64.

Adler, A. *Study of Organ Inferiority and Its Psychical Compensations.* New York: Nervous and Mental Disease Publishing Company, 1917.

Allport, Gordon. *The Nature of Prejudice.* Garden City, N.Y.: Doubleday-Anchor, 1958.

Ariès, Philippe. *Centuries of Childhood: A Social History of Family Life.* Translated by Robert Baldick. New York: Vintage Books, 1962.

Barker, R., B. Wright, L. Meyerson, and M. Gonick. *Adjustment to Physical Handicaps and Illness: A Survey of the Social Psychology of Physical Disability.* New York: Social Science Research Council, 1953. Bulletin 53.

Barocas, R. and P. Karely. "Effects of Physical Appearance on Social Responsiveness." *Psychological Reports* 31 (1972): 495–500.

Barocas, R. and F. Vance. "Physical Appearance and Personal Adjustment to Counseling." *Journal of Consulting and Clinical Psychology* 21 (1974): 96–100.

Becker, Howard S. *Outsiders: Studies in the Sociology of Deviance.* New York: Free Press, 1963.

Bem, Daryl. *Beliefs, Attitudes, and Human Affairs.* Belmont, Ca.: Brooks/Cole, 1970.

Berscheid, E., E. Walster, and G. Bohrenstedt. "The Happy Body: A Survey Report." *Psychology Today* 6 (1973): 119–31.

Beuf, Ann Hill. *Biting Off the Bracelet: A Study of Children in Hospitals.* 2nd ed. Philadelphia: University of Pennsylvania Press, 1989.

———. "The Stigmatization of Children." New York: World Health Organization, September 1979.

Beuf, Ann Hill and Judith Porter. "Children Coping with Impaired Appearance: Social and Psychological Influences." *General Hospital Psychiatry* 6 (Oct. 1984): 294–301.

Bruch, Hilde. *Eating Disorders: Anorexia, Obesity, and the Person Within.* New York: Basic Books, 1973.

Cash, T. and P. Begley. "Internal-External Control, Achievement Orientation, and Physical Attractiveness." *Psychology Reports* 38 (1976): 1205–06.

Cash, T., B. Gillen, and D. Burns. "Sexism and Beautyism in Personal Consultant Decision Making." *Journal of Applied Psychology* 62 (1977): 301–10.

Cash, T., J. Kehr, J. Polyson, and V. Freeman. "The Role of Physical Attractiveness in Peer Attribution of Psychological Disturbance." *Journal of Consulting and Clinical Psychology* 45 (1977): 987–93.

Centers, L. and R. Centers. "Peer Group Attitudes Toward the Amputee Child." *Journal of Social Psychology* 61 (1963): 127–32.

Christopherson, V. "Role Modification of the Disabled Male." *American Journal of Nursing* 68 (1968): 290–93.

Cleote, S. "I Speak for the African." *Life* 34 (1973): 111.

Coopersmith, S. *The Antecedents of Self-Esteem*. San Francisco: W. H. Freeman, 1967.

Davis, F. "Deviance Disavowal: The Management of Strained Interaction by the Visibly Handicapped." *Social Problems* 9 (1961): 120–32. Reprinted in F. Davis, *Illness, Interaction, and the Self*. Belmont, Ca.: Wadsworth, 1972. Pp. 130–58.

Dietz, Sheila, Madeleine Littman, and Brenda Bently. "Attribution of Responsibility for Rape: The Influences of Observer Empathy, Victim Resistance, and Victim Attractiveness." *Sociology of Sex Roles* 10 (Feb. 1984): 260–80.

Dion, Karen. "Physical Attractiveness and Evaluation of Children's Transgressions." *Journal of Personality and Social Psychology* 24 (1972): 207–13.

———. "What is Beautiful is Good." *Journal of Personality and Social Psychology* 24 (1972): 215–20.

Dixon, J. "Coping with Prejudice: Attitudes of Handicapped Persons Toward the Handicapped." *Journal of Chronic Disease* 30 (1977): 307–22.

Doob, H. and B. Ecker. "Stigma and Compliance." *Journal of Personality and Social Psychology* 14 (1970): 302–04.

Douglas, Helen Gahagan. *The Eleanor Roosevelt We Remember*. New York.

Dwyer, J. and J. Meyer. "Psychological Effects of Variation in Physical Appearance During Adolescence." *Adolescent* 3 (1968–1969): 353–58.

Erikson, Erik. *Childhood and Society*. 2nd ed., rev. New York: W. W. Norton, 1968.

Farina, A., J. Allen, and B. Saul. "The Role of the Stigmatized Person in Affecting Social Relationships." *Journal of Personality* 36 (1968): 169–82.

Fiedler, Leslie A. *Freaks: Myths and Images of the Secret Self*. New York; Simon and Schuster, 1978.

Fleishman, Jeffrey G. and Carol Cleveland. "Broken Children." *Allentown, Pa. Morning Call*, Nov. 1988, #35, 116, pp. 1, 4, 6, 8.

Fugita, S., T. Agie, I. Newman, and N. Walfish. "Attractiveness, Self Concept and a Methodological Note About Gaze." *Personality and Social Psychology Bulletin* 3 (1977): 240–43.

Goffman, Erving. *Stigma: Notes on the Management of Spoiled Identity*. Englewood Cliffs, N.J.: Prentice-Hall, 1963.

Goodman, N., S. Dornbusch, S. Robinson, and A. Hastorf. "Variant Reactions to Physical Disabilities." *American Sociological Review* 28 (1963): 429–35.

Greenleaf, Barbara Kaye. *Children Through the Ages*. New York: Barnes and Noble, 1978.

Grey, David and Richard Ashmore. "Biasing Influence on Sentencing: Characteristics of Simulated Sentencing." *Psychology Reports* 38, 1 (June 1976): 727–38.

Halperin, Jane. "The Emotional Aspects of N.F.: From the Beginning the Impact of Diagnosis." *Neurofibromatosis* (Winter 1988): 1, 7. New York: National Neurofibromatosis Association.

Hobfoll, Steven and Louis Pennerm. "Effect of Physical Attractiveness on Therapists' Initial Judgments of a Person's Self-Concept." *Journal of Consulting and Clinical Psychology* 46 (1978): 200–201.

Johnson, R. and L. Heal. "Private Employment Agency Responses to the Physically Handicapped." *Journal of Applied Rehabilitation Counseling* 7 (1976): 12–21.

Kleck, Robert. "Physical Stigma and Non-Verbal Cues Emitted in Face-to-Face Interaction." *Human Relations* 21 (1968): 19–28.

Kleck, R., H. Ono, and A. Hastorf. "Effects of Physical Deviance on Face-to-Face Interaction." *Human Relations* 19 (1966): 425–36.

Kitsuse, John I. "Societal Reaction to Deviant Behavior." *Social Problems* 9, 4 (Winter 1962): 247–56.

Kmiecik, Cynthia, Paula Mauser, and George Banzinger. "Attractiveness and Interpersonal Space." *Journal of Social Psychology* 108 (Aug. 1979): 277–78.

Kohn, M. *Social Class and Conformity: A Study in Values*. Homewood: Dorsey Press, 1969.

Landy, D. and H. Sigall. "Beauty is Talent: Task Evaluation as a Function of the Performer's Physical Attractiveness." *Journal of Personality and Social Psychology* 29 (1974): 299–304.

Lane, Lydia. "An Ugly Duckling Complex." *Los Angeles Times,* May 10, 1974.

Langer, E. J., *et al.* "Stigma, Staring, and Discomfort: A Novelty Stimulus Hypothesis." *Journal of Experimental Psychology* 12 (1976): 451–63.

Lefcourt, H. "Internal Versus External Control of Reinforcement. A Review." *Psychological Bulletin* 65 (1966): 206–20.

Lemert, Edwin M. *Social Pathology.* New York: McGraw-Hill, 1951.

Lenski, Gerhard and Jean Lenski. *Human Societies.* 4th. ed. New York: McGraw-Hill, 1982.

Lerner, Aaron and James Nordlund. "Vitiligo: What is it? Is it Important?" *JAMA* 239 (1978): 1183–89.

Let's Face It: A Network for People with Facial Disfigurement. Concord, Mass.: Let's Face It, 1988.

Levitt, L. and R. Kornhaber. "Stigma and Compliance: A Re-Examination." *Journal of Social Psychology* 18 (1977): 13–18.

Lewinski, R. and I. Kass. "Functional Disturbance Associated with Ichthyosis." *Journal of Psychology* 13 (1942): 173–77.

Liachowitz, Claire H. *Disability as a Social Construct: Legislative Roots.* Philadelphia: University of Pennsylvania Press, 1988.

Linton, Ralph. *The Study of Man.* New York: Appleton Century, 1936.

Lofland, John. *Deviance and Identity.* Englewood Cliffs, N.J.: Prentice-Hall, 1969.

MacGregor, Frances Cooke. *Transformation and Identity: The Face and Plastic Surgery.* Oak Grove, Ill.: Eterna Press, 1980.

———. *Facial Deformities and Plastic Surgery.* New York: Charles Thomas, 1953.

Mathes, Eugene. "The Effects of Physical Attractiveness on Behavior: A Test of the Self-Fulfilling Prophecy Theory." *Dissertation Abstracts International* (1974), 37, 5226.

Matza, David. *Delinquency and Drift.* New York: John Wiley, 1964.

McKelvie, S. and J. Mathews. "Effects of Physical Attractiveness and Favorableness of Character on Liking." *Psychological Reports* 38 (1976): 1223–30.

Menkes, John. *Textbook of Child Neurology.* Philadelphia: Lea and Febiger, 19XX.

Mercer, Janice, Henry Andrews, and Arthur Mercer. "The Effects of Physical Attractiveness and Disability on Client Ratings by Helping Professionals." *Journal of Applied Rehabilitation Counseling* 14 (1983): 41–45.

Miller, A. "The Role of Physical Attractiveness in Impression Formation." *Psychonomic Science* 19 (1970): 103–09.

———. "Social Perception and Internal/External Control." *Perceptual and Motor Skills* 30 (1970): 103–09.

Millman, Marcia. *Such a Pretty Face: Being Fat in America.* New York: W. W. Norton, 1980.

Money, J. and E. Pollet. "Studies in the Psychology of Dwarfism." *Journal of Pediatrics* 68 (1966): 391–96.

Murray, Joseph E., John Mulliken, Leonard Kapan, and Myron Belfer. "Twenty Year Experience in Maxillo-Craniofacial Surgery." *Annals of Surgery* 190, 3 (Sept. 1979): 320–21.

Neurofibromatosis 9, 2 (19xx) special issue.

New York Times, November 16, 1980, p. 22E.

Parsons, T. and E. Bales. *Family, Socialization, and Interaction Processes.* Glencoe, Ill.: Free Press, 1965.

Pearlin, L. J. and Carma Schooler. "The Structure of Coping." *Journal of Health and Social Behavior* 8 (1978): 2–21.

Pillavin, I., *et al.* "Costs, Diffusion, and the Stigmatized Victim." *Journal of Personality and Social Psychology* 32 (1975): 429–38.

Porter, Judith, Ann Hill Beuf, James Nordlund, and Aaron Lerner. "Personal Responses of Patients to Vitiligo." *Archives of Dermatology* 114 (1978): 1384–85.

———. "Social and Psychological Effects of Vitiligo." Paper presented at NIH Workshop on vitiligo, Washington, D.C., March 1977.

"Report Reveals Rise in Child Abuse Cases." Allentown, Pa., *Morning Call,* April 25, 1987.

Richardson, Stephen A., H. Goodman, A. Hastor, and S. Dornbusch. "Cultural Uniformity in Reaction to Physical Disability." *American Sociological Review* 26 (1961): 241–47.

Rogers-Salyer, Marcy, A. Gayle Jensen, and Christopher Borden. "Effects of Facial Deformities and Physical Attractiveness on Mother-Infant Bonding." In *Craniofacial Surgery. Proceedings of the First International Congress of the International Society of Cranio-Maxillo-Facial Surgery,* 1985.

Rosenzweig, S., E. Fleming, and H. Clarke. *Revised Scoring Manual for Rosenzweig Picture/Frustration Study.* New York: Journal Press, 1947.

Rosenzweig, S., E. Fleming, and L. Rosenzweig. "The Children's Form of the Rosenzweig Picture/Frustration Study." *Journal of Psychology* 26 (1948): 141–91.

Rotter, J. "Generalized Expectancies for Internal Versus External Control." *Journal of Consulting and Clinical Psychology* 34 (1970): 226–28.

Rubington, Earl and Martin S. Wineberg, eds. *Deviance: The Interactionist Perspective.* New York: Macmillan, 1987.

Salyer, Kenneth and Marcy Rogers-Salyer with Members of the Texas Craniofacial Center. *Craniofacial Deformity: A Booklet for Parents.* Dallas: Texas Foundation for Craniofacial Deformities.

Scheff, Thomas. *Being Mentally Ill.* Chicago: Aldine, 1966.

Schur, Edwin M. *Labeling Women Deviant: Gender, Stigma, and Social Control*. New York: Random House, 1984.
———. *The Politics of Deviance*. Englewood Cliffs, N.J.: Prentice-Hall, 1980.
Schwartz, J. and S. Abramonitz. "Effects of Female Client Physical Attractiveness on Clinical Judgment." *Psychotherapy: Theory, Research, and Practice* 15 (1978): 251–57.
Showalter, Elaine. *The Female Malady: Women, Madness, and English Culture, 1830–1890*. New York: Penguin, 1984.
Shuster, S., G. Fisher, E. Harris, and D. Binnell. "The Effects of Skin Diseases on Self-Image." *British Journal of Dermatology* 99 (1978): 18–19.
Siller, J., L. Ferguson, D. Vann, and B. Holland. "The Structure of Attitudes Toward the Physically Disabled.' The Disability Factor Scale: Amputation, Blindness, Cosmetic Conditions." *Proceedings of the 76th Annual Convention of the American Psychological Association* 3 (1978): 251–57.
Skolnick, Arlene. "The Myth of the 'Vulnerable Child.'" *Psychology Today* (Feb. 1978): 55–60, 65.
Sudnow, David. "Normal Crimes." *Social Problems* 12 (Winter 1965): 255–76.
Supersteim, Gary and Milton Budoff. "Effects of the Labels 'Mentally Retarded' and 'Retarded' on the Social Acceptability of Mentally Retarded Children." *American Journal of Mental Deficiency* 84 (1980): 596–601.
Taylor, S. and W. Reitz. *The Three Faces of Self-Esteem*. Department of Psychology, University of Western Ontario, Research Bulletin 80, 1968.
VanderKolk, C. J. "Physiological Measures as a Means of Assessing Reactions to the Disabled." *New Outlook for the Blind* 70 (1976): 101–03.
Ventimiglia, J. C. "Sex Roles and Chivalry: Some Conditions to Altruism." *Sociology of Sex Roles* 8 (Nov. 1982): 1107–22.
Whitlock, F. *Psychophysiological Aspects of Skin Disorder*. London: W. B. Saunders, 1976.
Wiseman, J. P. *The Lively Commerce*. New York: Signet Books, 1972.
Wolfgang, J. and A. Wolfgang. "Personal Space: An Unobtrusive Measure of Attitudes Toward the Physically Handicapped." *Proceedings of the 76th Annual Convention of the American Psychological Association* 3 (1978): 653–54.
Wright, Beatrice A. *Physical Disability: A Psychosocial Approach*. New York: Harper and Row, 1960. Second edition 1983.
Zelizer, Vivian A. *Pricing the Priceless Child: The Changing Social Value of Children*. New York: Basic Books, 1985.

Index

self-esteem, 18, 19, 20, 24, 74;
Coopersmith measure, ix
self-stigmatization, 10, 16, 19, 21, 24,
66, 83
self-fulfilling prophecy, 19
"Sesame Street," 107
severity, as factor in stigma, 23, 68,
84, 85
Showalter, Elaine, 32
Skolnick, Arlene, 75
social: distance, 13; factors in stigma,
8, 33–34, 44; resources, 20, 24, 60.
See also stigma, social nature of
socio-economic status. See wealth
sources of stigma: acquaintances and
peers, 47, 53; close friends and family, 47, 54; professionals, 47 (see also
medical establishment); strangers,
48
stereotypes, 13
stigma: defined, 3, 28; children and,
3; and label as deviant, 14; social
nature of, 10, 13, 17, 19, 20, 85
stigmatization, 1, 3, 6, 8, 14, 17, 19,
27, 39, 50, 108; non-verbal, 49;
prevention of, 64–65; stigmatizing

experiences, 81, 86; vulnerability to,
59. See also self-stigmatization
Sturges-Weber syndrome, 84

trivialization, 58, 84

universality, of definitions, 32
Updike, John, 84

value systems, 32, 33
Vance, F., 12
Ventimiglia, J.C., 18
visibility, 15, 23, 59, 65, 77, 85, 88–
89
vitiligo, ix, 2, 5, 51, 57, 61, 65, 71,
73–78, 81, 84, 85, 91–92

wealth: as coping resource, 22, 23; as
master status, 15
weight loss. See eating disorders
Wilson, Betsy, 113
withdrawal, as coping mechanism,
104
Wright, Beatrice A., 17
Weight Watchers, 38